Surgery
AND THE
Endocrine System

PHYSIOLOGIC RESPONSE TO SURGICAL TRAUMA—
OPERATIVE MANAGEMENT OF ENDOCRINE DYSFUNCTION

By JAMES D. HARDY, M.D., F.A.C.S.

Assistant Professor of Surgery
University of Tennessee Medical College

Illustrated

W. B. SAUNDERS COMPANY
Philadelphia & London
1952

COPYRIGHT, 1952, BY W. B. SAUNDERS COMPANY

COPYRIGHT UNDER THE INTERNATIONAL COPYRIGHT UNION

All rights reserved.
This book is protected by copyright.
No part of it may be duplicated or reproduced in any manner
without written permission from the publisher. Made in the
United States of America at the Press
of W. B. Saunders Company,
Philadelphia

TO MY WIFE

"THERE IS A CIRCUMSTANCE ATTENDING ACCIDENTAL INJURY WHICH DOES NOT BELONG TO DISEASE—NAMELY, THAT THE INJURY DONE HAS IN ALL CASES A TENDENCY TO PRODUCE THE DISPOSITION AND THE MEANS OF CURE."

John Hunter
1794

FOREWORD

This monograph by Dr. Hardy provides a rational basis for extending the care of the surgical patient. He has very aptly stated in his preface that the book attempts to clarify for the general surgeon the ways in which certain recent advances in physiology affect surgical care. It provides tangible evidence of the surgeon's continuing interest in the complete care of his patients.

The volume goes even further than this, for it summarizes certain trends in the surgical management of diseases of the endocrine organs. The volume covers a wide variety of subjects, many of which are closely interrelated, and all of which are of daily concern to the surgeon.

This is not a handbook of preoperative and postoperative care. It is, however, a volume which provides the physiologic basis for many types of surgical therapy. It gives further evidence of the abnormalities of function imposed by disease and injury. Certain of these circumstances are of a complex nature, but the author his presented his material as simply as possible.

Numerous of the subjects which Dr. Hardy has covered will require further intensive investigation before they are completely understood. He has, however, brought all available material together which can be accepted at this time, and this in itself is an achievement of real merit. His bibliographies are excellent.

In addition, he has in the presentation of his own investigations given us a clearer insight into many of these problems. He is to be congratulated on what he has achieved. Many years ago, William Mayo said that young men would do many things that older men would not attempt to do. Dr. Hardy's volume proves how true this statement is.

I. S. RAVDIN, M.D.

Philadelphia

PREFACE

The ability of man to survive injury is the foundation upon which the practice of surgery has been established. The extent of this capacity varies from one individual to another and even in the same individual from time to time. Logic and experience indicate that there must exist causes for these differences. The surgeon daily acknowledges the existence of such factors when he insists upon adequate preoperative nutrition, restoration of the normal blood volume, an anesthetic suited to the patient and aggressive postoperative care. Some of these causes are perhaps as fundamental as life itself, but many of the basic physiologic requirements fulfilled by previously empiric therapy are being identified.

Our first objective in writing this volume has been to outline the mechanisms by which the patient survives injury, and to attempt to clarify for the general surgeon ways in which certain recent advances in physiology affect surgical care. That is, we have endeavored to indicate the physiologic bases upon which intelligent management may enhance the capacity of the patient to withstand surgery. In taking this inventory, we have had to recognize the very considerable part which the endocrine organs play in mobilizing and transporting the metabolic reserves in an emergency. The metabolic processes of carbohydrates, proteins, fats, body fluids and antibodies are markedly influenced by the level of activity of one or more of the endocrine organs. In turn, the quality of the hormonal response to injury is affected by the preoperative state of nutrition. The supportive role of the hormones in stress is probably mediated through their influence on the activity of enzymes, which in turn regulate basic cytochemical reactions.

In Chapter 1, which is devoted to a resume of the alarm response, the pre-eminent roles of the adrenals, thyroid, and pituitary are sketched against the general background of the metabolic reaction to injury. Chapter 2 deals with the large influence which the hormones exercise in the regulation of the metabolism of body fluids and in shock. The ultimate significance of many of the postoperative alterations in body fluid composition and distribution is not known, but progress is often served by the systematic exposition of associated observations so that the experimental mosaic may be viewed in perspective. Chapter 3 concerns itself with some physiologic aspects of nutrition and with certain ways in which the nutritional status of the patient may affect his capacity to withstand trauma. Chapter 4 examines the physiologic consequences of prolonged bed rest and presents the rationale for early ambulation. Chapter 5 indicates briefly the importance of endocrinology in the fields of infection, tissue repair and regeneration, and neoplasia. Chapter 6 treats of endocrine therapy in surgical patients. These fields are still in their infancy.

Our second objective has been to present the facts and procedures which we consider most useful in the management of surgical diseases of the endocrine organs. A number of textbooks of endocrinology are available but, in general, these have been written by and for internists. There has appeared to be a real need for a work which would bring together those special endocrine problems which are of particular interest and importance to the general surgeon. Accordingly, Chapters 7 through 11 have been devoted to surgical problems related to the thyroid, parathyroids, pancreas, adrenals, pituitary, thymus, ovaries and testes. We have here emphasized material of practical value, and physiologic considerations have usually been presented only to clarify the newer diagnostic procedures. The management of complications has been stressed. No attempt has been made to portray in complete detail the operative technics for the various endocrine organs; these are available in appropriate operative manuals. Rather, the illustrations used are to indicate the broad outlines of operative approaches which the writer has found especially useful.

It gives the author great pleasure to acknowledge here the particular influence of the following teachers at the University of Pennsylvania Medical School, who have shown the way toward clinical proficiency and laboratory resourcefulness. These professors are Drs. I. S. Ravdin, Isaac Starr, Jonathan E. Rhoads, Julian Johnson and David L. Drabkin. This volume, which was written while the author was associated with the Harrison Department of Surgical Research, embodies indirect contributions by all.

The author wishes especially to thank the Director of the Department of Surgery at the University of Pennsylvania Medical School for his enthusiastic encouragement in all undertakings and for his unqualified generosity in making all materials and facilities available in the preparation of this work. The assistance of a Senior Damon Runyon Fellowship during part of the time this volume was in preparation is gratefully acknowledged.

We extend our sincere appreciation to the staff of the W. B. Saunders Company for their consideration and constructive editing.

Finally, the author expresses his deepest gratitude to Miss Florence V. Conway for her conscientious typing of the manuscript.

JAMES D. HARDY

Memphis
March, 1952

CONTENTS

1. THE ALARM REACTION IN THE SURGICAL PATIENT: GENERAL
   ENDOCRINE RELATIONSHIPS 1

   Outline of the Alarm Syndrome 1
   Functions of the Adrenal Cortex in Stress 3
   The Thyroid Gland in Stress 7
   Endocrine Interrelationships 7
   The Function of Other Endocrine Glands in Stress 8
   The Mechanism of Action of Hormones 8
   Practical Implications of the Alarm Response 9

2. METABOLIC ASPECTS OF BODY FLUID REGULATION AND OF SHOCK 15

   Fluid and Electrolyte Metabolism 15
   Changes in Fluid and Electrolyte Metabolism Following Major
     Surgical Procedures 18
   The Relation of Endocrines to Abnormal Fluid Deposits 22
   Metabolic Aspects of Shock 23

3. THE DYNAMICS OF NUTRITION: THE RELATION OF NUTRITION TO AN
   ADEQUATE RESPONSE TO TRAUMA 27

   Protein Metabolism in Stress Conditions 27
   Specific Endocrine Effects of Nitrogen Metabolism 27
   Factors in Lipid Metabolism 29
   Endocrine Influences in Carbohydrate Metabolism 30
   Vitamine-Endocrine Relationships 31
   Ways in Which Inadequate Nutrition Reduces Surgical Success .. 32
   The Adequate Diet 35

4. THE PHYSIOLOGIC BASIS OF EARLY AMBULATION: NOTES ON
   CONVALESCENCE 43

   Background of Early Ambulation in the United States 43
   Experimental Data in Support of Early Ambulation 44
   The Metabolic Effects of Prolonged Immobilization 45
   Muscular Strength and Circumference of the Extremities ... 46
   Postural Hemodynamics 47
   The Desire to Get Well 48

5. THE ENDOCRINOLOGY OF SURGICAL INFECTIONS, THERMAL BURNS,
   TISSUE REPAIR AND NEOPLASIA 51

   Surgical Infections 51
   Thermal Burns 51
   The Effects of Hormones on Tissue Repair and Regeneration . 52
   The Endocrinology of Neoplasia 53

6. ENDOCRINE THERAPY IN SURGICAL PATIENTS 59

    Absolute and Relative Adrenocortical Insufficiency in Patients
      coming to Surgery 59
    Management of Drug Sensitivities, Including Exfoliative Dermatitis 62
    Management of the Diabetic Patient Subjected to Surgery 62
    Hormonal Therapy in Advanced Malignancy 63
    Use of Testosterone to Increase Nitrogen Retention 66
    Posterior Pituitary Extracts 66

7. THE THYROID GLAND 69

    Anatomy and Embryology 69
    Pathology of the Thyroid Gland 72
    Management of Toxic Goiter 78

8. HYPERPARATHYROIDISM 99

    Physiology of the Parathyroids 99
    Pathologic Lesions in Hyperparathyroidism 100
    The Diagnosis of Primary Hyperparathyroidism 101
    Management of Primary Hyperparathyroidism 104

9. FUNCTIONING TUMORS OF THE ISLAND OF LANGERHANS 111

    Historical Considerations 111
    Pathology of Islet Cell Tumors 112
    The Diagnosis of Hyperinsulinism 113
    Surgical Management of Organic Hyperinsulinism 115

10. THE ADRENAL GLANDS: SURGICAL CONSIDERATIONS 119

    Adrenal Cortical Tumors and Hyperplasia 119
    Adrenalectomy for Essential Hypertension 128
    Functioning Tumors of the Adrenal Medulla (Pheochromocytoma) 128

11. THE PITUITARY, THYMUS, AND GONADS 137

    Tumors of the Pituitary 137
    Diseases of the Thymus Gland 139
    Functioning Tumors of the Ovary 140
    Tumors of the Testis 141

INDEX 143

CHAPTER 1

THE ALARM REACTION IN THE SURGICAL PATIENT:
General Endocrine Relationships

The concept that the organism reacts to emergency situations with highly integrated metabolic activities is not new. In 1914 Cannon published his investigations on the emergency function of the adrenal medulla in which he showed that emotional stimuli could release a substance which prepared the animal for flight or defense. In 1932 Cuthbertson in Great Britain described his classic observations on the prolonged alterations in metabolism produced by fractures of the long bones, and these studies illuminated avenues of research which are constantly being extended. A few years later Rudolf Schoenheimer and his associates, on the basis of their epic studies of fatty acid metabolism using the isotope deuterium as a tracer, enunciated the theory that the materials constituting the body tissues are continuously being utilized and excreted or restored to the common metabolic pool. This concept of the *dynamic state of body constituents* has since been amply confirmed.

It was against this background that Hans Selye, through extensive personal investigation and a unique perception of the integration of hitherto loosely correlated facts, formulated his now widely accepted theories of the "alarm syndrome" and the "processes of adaptation."

OUTLINE OF THE ALARM SYNDROME

When the patient is subjected to trauma, epinephine is promptly released through stimulation of the adrenal medulla. This produces the following well known sympathomimetic effects: a rise in general blood pressure and an increase in the force and output of the heart; hyperglycemia, resulting from the mobilization of carbohydrate from the labile stores in the liver and insuring an adequate supply of fuel; an increased oxygen carrying capacity of the blood due to the discharge of red cells from the spleen; bronchiolar dilatation and an increased rate and depth of respiration; and a shortened coagulation time of the blood. The evidence indicates that at the same time epinephrine stimulates the anterior pituitary to release increased amounts of adrenocorticotrophic hormone (ACTH) and, very likely, of thyroid stimulating hormone (TSH) into the blood stream. These two hormones in turn effect an increased activity of the adrenal cortex and the thyroid, respectively. Sayers and Sayers have shown that, in cats, within minutes following the onset of stress there is an increased rate of secretion of ACTH. This, with its effect of increasing adrenocortical activity, is exceedingly important in enabling the organism to withstand acute and prolonged stress.

While the increased activity of the adrenal cortex can be determined by the quantitative measurement of certain of its fractions excreted in the urine, there is a simpler and clinically more useful method for estimating

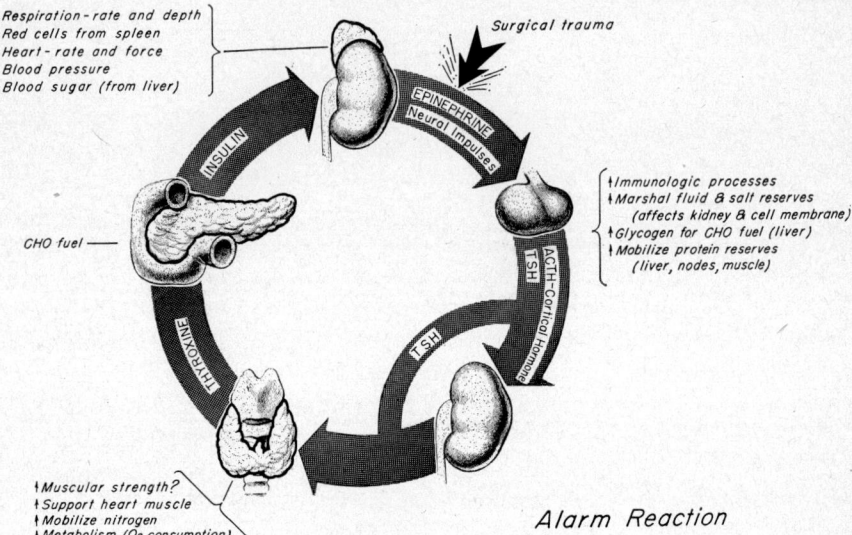

Fig. 1. The stress imposed by anesthesia and operation results in neural impulses and a release of epinephrine which stimulate an increased secretion of ACTH by the anterior pituitary. The resulting cycle of events is indicated in the diagram. It is to be noted that the alarm response is essentially an acceleration of ordinary physiologic processes. This response may be mediated through hormonal influences on rates of enzymatic activity.

changes in the level of adrenocortical activity. Thorn and his associates have developed the use of the total eosinophil count for this purpose. Briefly, when adrenocortical activity increases, the total eosinophil count decreases; and as the increased adrenocortical activity subsides, the total eosinophil count again rises. It is important to make control eosinophil counts preoperatively, since this value varies widely in different individuals. Changes in the postoperative period are then expressed as percentages of the preoperative level. Following a major surgical procedure the total eosinophil count frequently falls to zero and may remain there for twenty-four hours, after which it usually returns to normal or above normal values over the course of the next few days. In our experience, patients in whom the eosinophil count does not fall following trauma are apt to have a turbulent postoperative course.

FUNCTIONS OF THE ADRENAL CORTEX IN STRESS

The steroids secreted by the adrenal cortex have far reaching effects on widely separated phases of physiologic response. The functions of these hormones are inseparably interlocked with those of the pituitary, thyroid, pancreas, liver and other organs. The adrenal cortex has an important role in protein metabolism, but this role cannot be separated from its part in glucose metabolism. Likewise, lipid mobilization and

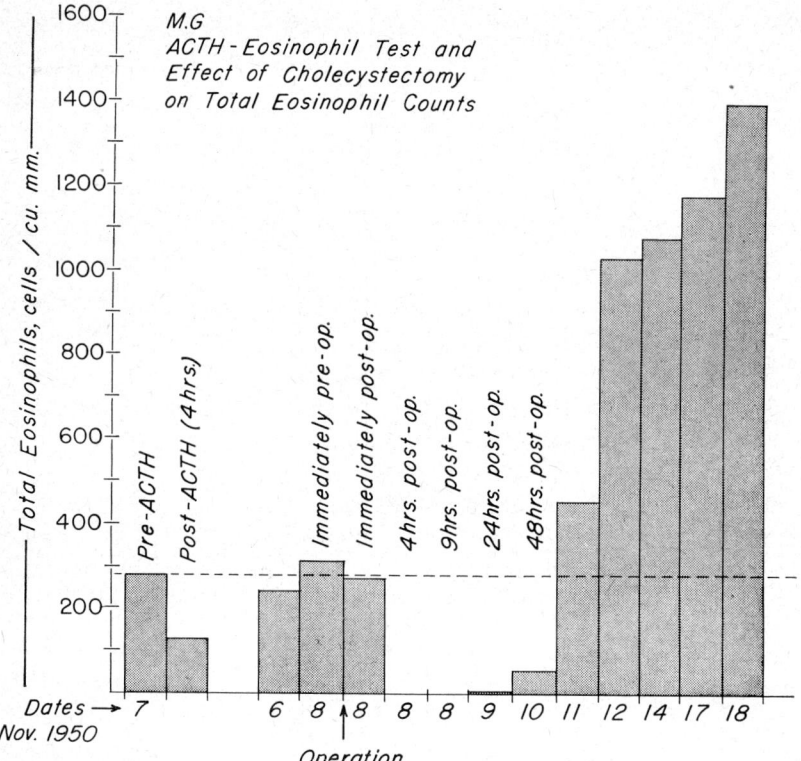

Fig. 2. The effect of operation in increasing adrenocortical activity is indicated by the fall in the total eosinophil count to zero within four hours following cholecystectomy. On the third postoperative day the eosinophil count had regained its preoperative level, and on the tenth postoperative day it was four times the preoperative level. There is evidence to suggest that rates of certain metabolic activities are subnormal during this period of high eosinophil counts (Hardy, J. D., unpublished data). The preoperative ACTH-eosinophil test indicates a normal adrenocortical reserve.

deposition in the liver is augmented in stress, a process which is diminished by adrenalectomy (Berman and associates).

The vital role of the adrenocortical steroids in preserving the normal volumes, distribution and electrolytic composition of body fluids has long been recognized. To meet emergency needs, the secretion of these hormones in increased amounts effects changes in fluid and electrolyte metabolism. For example, the urinary excretion of sodium, chloride and water is diminished in the early postoperative period, while the excretion of potassium is increased. This has been correlated with an increase in adrenocortical activity (Hardy; Johnson and associates).

The adrenal steroids have recently been shown to have a striking effect on bacterial infection. Kass, Ingbar and Finland found that cortisone

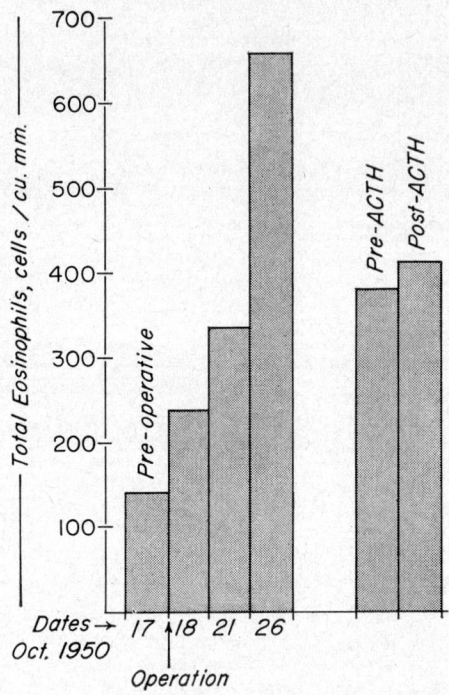

Fig. 3. The response of the total eosinophil count to operation in this patient is in marked contrast to that exhibited by the control patient in Figure 2, who had a cholecystectomy. Instead of diminishing following adrenalectomy, the total eosinophil count increased. Moreover, the ACTH-eosinophil count done one month later indicated an absence of significant adrenocortical reserve. These data are typical of those found in patients whose adrenal tissue has been almost completely removed at operation (This patient, T.C., was operated upon by Dr. Harold A. Zintel.)

abolished the symptoms and fever in patients with lobar pneumonia, even in the presence of a persistently positive blood culture. Dougherty, Chase and White demonstrated that a single injection of ACTH or adrenocortical extract (ACE) in hyperimmunized rabbits resulted in a rise in circulating antibodies within six hours. The response to ACTH was absent after adrenalectomy. Such studies promise a more profound understanding of the relationships between bacteria and the immunologic response of the host.

The exact role which the adrenal steroids exercise in the regulatory mechanism of the clotting process is obscure, but recent work indicates that ACTH and cortisone shorten the clotting and bleeding time (Cosgriff and associates).

The Steroids of the Adrenal Cortex

The known fractions of the adrenocortical secretion are numerous and others will doubtless be identified in the near future. At present at least twenty-seven steroids have been isolated in crystalline form from the adrenal glands of animals and their structural formulae have been determined, but the physiologic activities of only a few of these steroids have been studied carefully in human beings. This discussion will be limited to certain representative compounds which have an important role in supporting the response to stress.

Desoxycorticosterone (DOCA). This compound causes a marked retention of sodium, chloride and water and an increased urinary excretion of potassium. It has no effect on carbohydrate metabolism or on the pigmentation of Addison's disease. When administered in chronic adrenal insufficiency, it restores the normal electrolyte balance, increases the circulating blood volume, and raises the blood pressure.

11-Dehydro-17-hydroxycorticosterone (Compound E; Cortisone). This compound has a marked effect on carbohydrate metabolism. It promotes glycogen storage in the liver, increases blood sugar and prevents hypoglycemia. Cortisone also has an effect on fluid and salt metabolism; in some patients this effect appears adequate to maintain the integrity of these constituents in the absence of adrenal tissue.

17-Hydroxycorticosterone (Compound F). This steroid is similar to cortisone in its action. It has a considerable effect on carbohydrate metabolism, but it also increases the urinary excretion of sodium and produces a negative sodium balance.

The action of these compounds can be correlated with their structural formulae. For example, compounds with an oxygen atom at C-11 exercise a marked effect on carbohydrate metabolism. The presence of a 17-hydroxyl group causes the hormone to induce a negative sodium balance, and compounds without the 17-hydroxyl group exercise a salt-retaining effect.

Relation Between "Corticoids" and "17-Ketosteroids"

In addition to compounds such as those above, which are loosely termed "corticoids," there is another group of steroids secreted by the adrenal cortex and the testes termed "androgens" which cause nitrogen retention and an increased somatic growth. Testosterone is an androgen and it is similar in activity to those androgens secreted by the adrenal cortex. The androgens generally contain nineteen carbon atoms and the corticoids contain twenty-one carbon atoms. So far as is known, neither the corticoids nor the androgens are precursors of each other, though they may be shown to be derived from modifications of the same parent substance. (Cholesterol is believed by some to be the precursor of most steroids.)

In general, the androgenic substances break down into products which are measured grossly in the urine as "17-ketosteroids." The C-21 compounds (compounds E, F, A, B, etc.) break down into products excreted

TABLE 1
URINARY CORTICOIDS VS. URINARY 17-KETOSTEROIDS*
(Modified from Engstrom)

	CORTICOIDS	17-KETOSTEROIDS
Origin	Adrenal cortex	Adrenal cortex and testes
Number of carbon atoms in precursors	21	19
Examples of precursors	Compounds A, B, E, F, and desoxycorticosterone	Testosterone and adrenal androgens
Normal daily excretion	0.12 to 0.3 mg./24 hrs. in both sexes (Talbot)	Men, 6 to 25 mg. (avg. 14) Women, 5 to 17 mg. (avg. 10)
Metabolic action of precursors	Influence carbohydrate, protein and fluid metabolism	Promote nitrogen retention, muscular strength and weight gain
Effect of trauma on excretion	Increased	Less consistently increased

* Certain generalizations are employed.

in the urine and measured quantitatively as corticoids. The normal daily excretion of corticoids is about the same for males as for females, and is about 0.12 to 0.34 mg. per twenty-four hours as determined by the method of Talbot. (These values vary according to the method used for analysis.) The excretion of these substances may be enormously increased in the presence of adrenocortical tumors. The daily urinary excretion of 17-ketosteroids, however, is greater in men than in women because of the added increment from the testes in males. The average value is about 14 mg. in men and 10.2 mg. in women. Children present lower levels of excretion, depending upon their age. Those under seven excrete about 1.3 mg. per twenty-four hours (Engstrom). The 17-ketosteroid excretion also may be greatly increased in certain types of adrenocortical overactivity. It is often diminished in the presence of malnutrition, infections and hepatic disease.

THE THYROID GLAND IN STRESS

The established clinical observation that hypothyroid patients may be poor operative risks has been clarified experimentally. For example, the heart of a hypothyroid patient cannot respond normally to the emergency stimulus of epinephrine (Hoffman, Hoffman and Talesnik). Furthermore, thyroxine influences cellular oxygen consumption, a function which may be mediated through its effect on cytochrome C (Drabkin). Thus, since an increase in the general level of metabolism would appear to be helpful in enabling the patient to withstand trauma, it has seemed probable that the level of thyroid activity would be found to be increased in stress states. That this did in fact obtain was suggested by Cuthbertson's demonstration of an increased metabolic rate following injury. However, many factors influence the basal metabolic rate and until radioactive iodine became available for tracer studies of thyroid physiology an increased level of thyroid activity following operation and other stress conditions was not demonstrated.

Soffer and his associates had shown that epinephrine increased to a significant degree the blood level of thyrotropic hormone in normal, thyroidectomized or adrenalectomized animals, and Rawson and his colleagues had reported that the administration of epinephrine caused an increased discharge of iodine from, and a heightening of the epithelium of, the thyroid gland in rats. Carrying this type of experiment a bit further, Leblond and his associates showed that stress increased the pituitary secretion of thyrotropin and that this resulted in an increase in thyroid activity which was doubtful after one to three days, definite after seven days, maximal at twenty-six days, but absent after forty days. Similarly, Williams, Jaffe and Kemp concluded that various types of stress resulted in the release of an increased amount of thyrotropin by the pituitary body. This was followed by an increased production of thyroid hormone, but at the same time there was an increase in the rate at which the body tissues utilized thyroxine.

These studies, made with radioiodine as a tracer, help clarify previous observations that the serum protein-bound iodine level (presumably representing circulating thyroxine) does not change following operations which do not involve resection of the thyroid gland. Although thyroxine is being formed more rapidly following stress, it is at the same time being utilized in increased amounts by the tissues, resulting in little net change in the serum concentration of this hormone. Finally, Perry and Gemmell have reported a marked and sudden increase in the urinary excretion of iodine following operation, which again suggests that the metabolism of iodine and presumably of thyroxine is altered following trauma.

ENDOCRINE INTERRELATIONSHIPS

It is evident from the foregoing discussion that the endocrines form a closely integrated system which regulates the nature and extent of a vast number of metabolic activities. As knowledge increases we find that in many instances the maximum effectiveness of a particular hormone is dependent upon the presence of another hormone. For example, Hoffman, Hoffman and Talesnik have demonstrated that the adrenocortical hormones are necessary for thyroxine to exert its usual stimulation of cellular oxygen consumption. Also, the full effect of thyroxine in mobilizing muscle nitrogen in stress is dependent upon the presence of adrenocortical hormones (White and Dougherty).

There appears to exist a correlation between the level of thyroid activity and the level of adrenocortical activity, but the precise definition of

TABLE 2
REFLECTIONS ON FEVER: IS FEVER A COMPONENT OF THE ALARM RESPONSE?

1. Fever accompanies sterile trauma.
2. Fever is abetted by a decrease in heat elimination through a limitation of sweat formation.
3. Following trauma the tendency to sweat appears to be diminished (Hardy, J. D., unpublished observations).
4. A decline in fever is frequently associated with "spontaneous" sweating.
5. The absence of fever in severe infections is often an unfavorable prognostic sign.
6. *Tentative hypothesis:* Trauma results in a central suppression of sweating. The decreased heat elimination which ensues results in fever. The increased heat thus made available acts physically to accelerate rates of metabolic activity. Thus, it is possible that fever in moderation is beneficial in enabling the organism to withstand trauma.

this relationship remains to be formulated. While the injection of epinephrine increases the level of activity of both the thyroid and the adrenal cortex, Hardy, Riegel and Erisman have shown that the parenteral administration of either ACTH or cortisone results in a decrease in the serum level of protein-bound iodine. Moreover, there may be a decreased uptake of radioiodine by the thyroid gland following such therapy. Conversely, the clinical picture of the crisis of Addison's disease has frequently been compared with that of thyroid storm.

THE FUNCTION OF OTHER ENDOCRINE GLANDS IN STRESS

The functions of the islands of Langerhans, the parathyroids and the gonads in stress have yet to be evaluated in man.

THE MECHANISM OF ACTION OF HORMONES

It is increasingly evident that most hormonal actions will eventually find their proximate explanation in appropriate enzyme systems, but as yet the outlines of such control are still dim. Hormones do not initiate new types of cellular activity; they merely influence the rate at which these proceed. Since it is now recognized that cellular function is based on underlying chemical transformations, it is necessary to assume that through enzyme systems the hormones influence these reactions in cells

(Long). An example of this type of relationship is the finding by Price, Cori and Colowick that an anterior pituitary hormone and insulin exert at least a part of their physiologic action by regulating the rate of the hexokinase reaction which is a major step in the formation of glycogen from glucose.

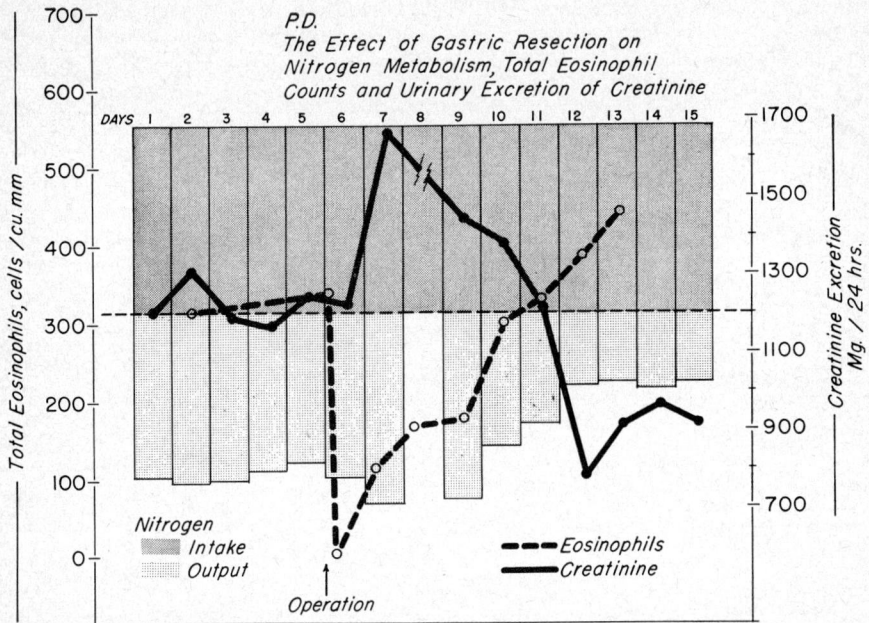

Fig. 4. Certain metabolic alterations following trauma. Changes in the total eosinophil counts and in the urinary excretion of nitrogen and creatinine are presented. The total eosinophil count fell to zero within four hours following operation, returning to and exceeding the preoperative level on the fifth postoperative day. The urinary excretion of creatinine was increased by trauma, a common finding following large operations (Hardy, J. D., unpublished data).

After operation there was a prompt increase in the urinary nitrogen excretion, followed by a retention of nitrogen which coincided with a fall in the creatinine excretion and a rise in the total eosinophil counts. The curve for creatinine excretion was closely paralleled by the curves representing changes in the urinary excretion of corticoids and 17-ketosteroids (Hardy, J., Richardson, E., and Dohan, C.: To be published).

The enzymes themselves are protein in nature, at times in association with other compounds. They are usually quite specific in their action, but this action is influenced by a wide variety of physical and chemical conditions. A large number of enzymes have been studied, among them being such familiar ones as amylase, lipase and trypsin, and a great many others will surely be identified. Indeed, enzyme studies are rapidly assuming a central position in organic chemistry.

PRACTICAL IMPLICATIONS OF THE ALARM RESPONSE

In order for the patient to have an adequate response to stress and thus insure a successful operation, his pituitary-thyroid-adrenal axis and its supporting organs must be essentially intact. A failure of any link in this chain jeopardizes the integrity of the total response to stress. As we have seen, the patient who has pituitary insufficiency (panhypopituitarism), thyroid insufficiency (myxedema) or adrenal insufficiency (Addison's disease) cannot react adequately to the trauma of anesthesia and operation. Fortunately, such states can be diagnosed preoperatively. The absence of a fall in the total eosinophil count following the administration of epinephrine indicates poor pituitary function, provided a nor-

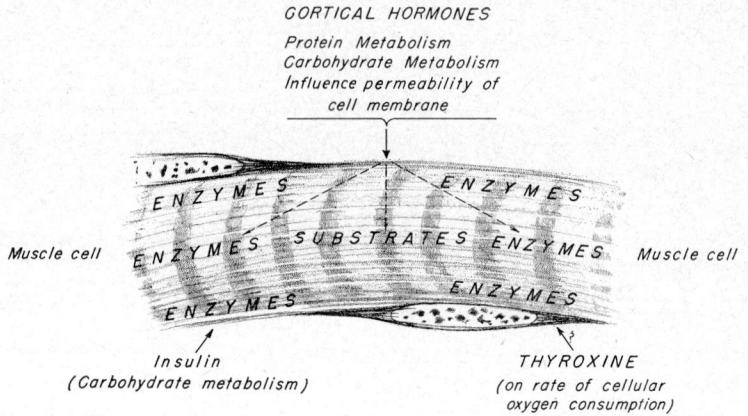

Possible Site of Action of Hormones

Fig. 5. Possible site of hormonal action. There is evidence that hormones may exert their influence on rates of enzymatic activity along the cell membrane. However, if one conceives of the hormonal effects on permeability as affecting also the permeability of intracellular components (in addition to the cell membrane), the surfaces available for contacts between hormones and enzymes are enormously increased (Dr. William C. Stadie). The influence of the adrenocortical C-21 steroids on the rates of transfer of water and electrolytes across the cell membrane is especially illustrative of permeability effects.

mal response to ACTH is obtained. If the total eosinophil count does not fall following the administration of ACTH, the adrenal cortex is at fault (Thorn). Such patients should receive appropriate supportive therapy.

A number of studies have shown that the magnitude of many phases of the alarm response is diminished in the presence of malnutrition. This is in keeping with the abundant clinical evidence that if the process of weight loss can be reversed and the patient gain even a few pounds he is a much better operative risk.

The effects of the endocrine system on fluid and electrolyte metabolism in the normal person and in the postoperative patient must receive consideration in planning replacement therapy. Obviously, it is unwise to load the patient with sodium chloride in the early postoperative period when the net effect of adrenocortical hormones on the kidney tubules is to decrease the excretion of this salt. The moderate hypochloremia, hypokalemia and an increased serum bicarbonate which occur in the early postoperative period may merely be a result of the transfer of water out of the cells. In this case, such changes in electrolyte concentration may be looked upon as a normal response to stress and require no correction.

Finally, the process of convalescence, of "getting well," has scarcely been explored. True, many able investigators have devoted their best efforts to this problem, but adequate methods were not theirs to command. The concept of reaction and of adaptation to a particular stress may afford the framework within which we can appreciate why a patient is less hard hit by a second operation than by the first, provided sufficient time has elapsed in the interim. The proper spacing of staged operations deserves investigation. The correlation of urinary steroid excretion with the clinical course in such patients may supply some of these answers, and such work is in progress in our laboratory.

The specific functions of the endocrines in such fields as growth, tissue repair and regeneration, and neoplasia are certain to be more carefully defined, and such knowledge will ultimately be of great assistance to the practicing surgeon in the daily care of his patients.

REFERENCES

Baldwin, E.: Dynamic Aspects of Biochemistry. New York, The Macmillan Company, 1947.
Barker, S. B.: Metabolic functions of the endocrine system. Ann. Rev. Physiol., 11:45, 1949.
Berman, D., Sylvester, M., Hay, E. C., and Selye, H.: The adrenal and early hepatic regeneration. Endocrinology, 41:258, 1947.
Cannon, W. B.: The emergency function of the adrenal medulla in pain and the major emotions. Am. J. Physiol., 33:356, 1914.
Chase, J. H., White, A., and Dougherty, T. F.: Enhancement of circulating antibody concentration by adrenal cortical hormones. J. Immunol., 52:101, 1946.
Cheng, C., Sayers, G., Goodman, L. S., and Swinyard, C. A.: Discharge of adrenocorticotrophic hormone in the absence of neural connections between the pituitary and hypothalamus. Am. J. Physiol., 158:45, 1949.
Coller, F. A., Campbell, K. N., Vaughan, H. H., Iob, L. V., and Moyer, C. A.: Postoperative salt intolerance. Ann. Surg., 119:533, 1944.
Conn, J. W., Vogel, W. C., Louis, L. H., and Fajans, S. S.: Serum cholesterol: a probable precursor of adrenal cortical hormones; in American Association for the Advancement of Science, Section on Medical Sciences: Pituitary-Adrenal Function. Washington, The association, 1951.
Cooper, D. R., Iob, V., and Coller, F. A.: Response to parenteral glucose of normal kidneys and of kidneys of postoperative patients. Ann. Surg., 129:1, 1949.
Cope, O., Nathanson, I. T., Rourke, N., and Wilson, H.: Metabolic observations. Ann. Surg., 117:937, 1943.
Cosgriff, S. W., Stuart, W., Diefenbach, A. F., and Vogt, W., Jr.: Hypercoagulability of the blood associated with ACTH and cortisone therapy. Am. J. Med., 9:752, 1950.
Cuthbertson, D. P.: Observations on the disturbance of metabolism produced by injury to the limbs. Quart. J. Med., 1:233, 1932.
———, McGirr, J. L., and Robertson, J. M. S.: The effect of fracture of bone on the metabolism of the rat. Quart. J. Exper. Physiol., 29:13, 1939.
Deane, H. W.: Physiological regulation of the zona glomerulosa of the rat's adrenal cortex, as revealed by cytochemical observations; in American Association for the

Advancement of Science, Section on Medical Sciences: Pituitary-Adrenal Function. Washington, The association, 1951.

—— and Greep, R. O.: Cytochemical study of adrenal cortex in hypo- and hyperthyroidism. Endocrinology, 41:243, 1947.

Dougherty, T. F., Chase, J. H., and White, A.: Demonstration of antibodies in lymphocytes. Proc. Soc. Exper. Biol. & Med., 58:135, 1945.

—— and White, A.: Adrenal cortical secretion and lymphoid tissue. J. Lab. & Clin. Med., 32:584, 1947.

Drabkin, D. L.: The effect of thyroidectomy and thiouracil on cytochrome C metabolism and liver regeneration. Federation Proc., 7:151, 1948.

Ehrich, W. E., and Seifter, J.: Role played by salivary glands in alarm reaction. Arch. Path., 45:239, 1948.

Engstrom, W. W.: Nature and significance of neutral steroids in human urine in normal and abnormal states. Yale J. Biol. & Med., 21:19, 1948–49.

Forbes, A. P., Donaldson, E. C., Reifenstein, E. C., Jr., and Albright, F.: Effect of trauma and disease on urinary 17-ketosteroid excretion in man. J. Clin. Endocrinol., 7:264, 1947.

Gemmell, J. P., and Perry, W. F.: The effect of ACTH and surgical operations on iodine excretion. Canad. J. Research, 28:147, 1950.

Gordon, A. S., and Charipper, H. A.: Endocrine system and hemopoiesis. Ann. New York Acad. Sci., 48:615, 1947.

Green, J. D., and Harris, G. W., Jr.: Neurovascular link between neurohypophysis and adenohypophysis. J. Endocrinol., 5:136, 1946.

Hardy, J. D.: The adrenal cortex and postoperative gastrointestinal secretions. Surgery, 29:517, 1951.

——: The role of adrenal cortex in the postoperative retention of salt and water. Ann. Surg., 132:189, 1950.

——, Riegel, C., and Erisman, E. P.: Experience with protein bound iodine (PBI): effect of ACTH and cortisone on thyroid function. Am. J. M. Sc., 219:581, 1950.

Harris, G. W.: Blood vessels of rabbit's pituitary gland, and significance of pars and zona tuberalis. J. Anat., 81:343, 1947.

Heard, R. D. H., and Sobel, H.: A colorimetric method for the estimation of reducing steroids. J. Biol. Chem., 165:687, 1946.

——, Sobel, H., and Venning, E. H.: The neutral lipid-soluble reducing substances of urine as an index of adrenocortical function. Ibid., 699.

Hellman, L., Weston, R. E., Escher, D. J. W., and Leiter, L.: Effect of adrenocorticotrophin on renal hemodynamics and uric acid clearance. Federation Proc., 7:52, 1948.

Hemphill, R. E., and Reiss, M.: Regulation of endogenous cortin production. Endocrinology, 41:17, 1947.

Hoffman, F., Hoffman, E. J., and Talesnik, J.: Effect of thyroid hormone on mammalian heart. Am. J. Physiol., 148:689, 1947.

——, Hoffman, E. J., and Talesnik, J.: The influence of thyroxine and adrenal cortical extract on the oxygen consumption of adrenalectomized rats. J. Physiol., 107:251, 1948.

Holtorff, A. F., and Kock, F. C.: The colorimetric estimation of 17-ketosteroids and their applcation to urine extracts. J. Biol. Chem., 135:377, 1940.

Johnson, H. T., Conn, J. W., Iob, V., and Coller, F. A.: Postoperative salt retention and its relation to increased adrenal cortical function. Ann. Surg., 132:374, 1950.

Kass, E. H., Ingbar, S. H., and Finland, M.: Effects of adrenocorticotropic hormone in pneumonia: clinical, bacteriological, and serological studies. Ann. Int. Med., 33:1081, 1950.

Keller, A. D., and Breckenridge, C. G.: Retention of normal insulin tolerance and adrenal cortex after extirpation of hypophysial stalk in dog. Am. J. Physiol., 150:222, 1947.

Kimeldorf, D. J., and Soderwall, A. L.: Ovarian hormones and adrenal cortex changes induced in the adrenal cortical zones by ovarian hormones. Endocrinology, 41:21, 1947.

Leblond, C. P., Gross, J.: Peacock, W., and Evans, R. D.: Metabolism of radioiodine in the thyroids of rats exposed to high or low temperatures. Am. J. Physiol., *140:* 671, 1944.

Leblond, C. P., and Hoff, H. E.: Comparison of cardiac and metabolic actions of thyroxine, thyroxine derivatives, and dinitrophenol in thyroidectomized rats. Ibid., *141:*32, 1944.

Leindorfer, A., Arana, R., and Hack, M. H.: Hyperglycemia induced by action of adrenalin on central nervous system. Am. J. Physiol., *150:*588, 1947.

Long, C. N. H.: Conditions associated with secretion of adrenal cortex. Federation Proc., *6:*461, 1947.

——: Factors regulating the adrenal cortical secretion; in American Association for the Advancement of Science, Section on Medical Sciences: Pituitary-Adrenal Function. Washington, The association, 1951.

Ludewig, S., and Chanutin, A.: The adrenal cholesterol and ascorbic acid contents after injury. Endocrinology, *41:*135, 1947.

Marrian, G. E.: Some aspects of intermediary metabolism of steroid hormones (Harvey Lecture). Bull. New York Acad. Med., *15:*27, 1939.

Mason, H. L., and Engstrom, W. W.: The 17-ketosteroids: their origin, determination and significance. Physiol. Rev., *30:*32, 1950.

Means, J. H.: The Thyroid and Its Diseases. 2d ed. Philadelphia, J. B. Lippincott Company, 1948, p. 103.

Meyer, A. E.: Inositol, a constituent of thyroid gland, effect on perfused rabbit's heart. Proc. Soc. Exper. Biol. & Med., *62:*111, 1946.

Overman, R. R., Davis, A. K., and Bass, A. C.: Effect of cortisone and DCA on Na^{24} transport in adrenalectomized dogs. Federation Proc., *10:*100, 1951.

Paschkis, K. E., Cantarow, A., Eberhard, T., and Boyle, D.: Thyroid function in the alarm reaction. Proc. Soc. Exper. Biol. & Med., *73:*116, 1950.

Perry, W. F., and Gemmell, J. P.: The effect of surgical operations on the excretion of iodine, corticosteroids and uric acid. Canad. J. Research, *27:*320, 1949.

Price, W. H., Cori, C. F., and Colowick, S. P.: Effect of anterior pituitary extract and insulin on hexokinase reaction. J. Biol. Chem., *160:*633, 1945.

Rawson, R. W., and McArthur, J. W.: Radioiodine, its use as tool in study of thyroid physiology. J. Clin. Endocrinol., *7:*235, 1947.

Sayers, G.: The adrenal cortex and hemostasis. Physiol. Rev., *30:*241, 1950.

—— and Sayers, M. A.: The pituitary-adrenal system. Recent Progr. Hormone Research, *2:*81, 1948.

Sayers, M. A., Sayers, G., and Woodbury, L. A.: Assay of adrenocorticotrophic hormone by adrenal ascorbic acid-depletion method. Endocrinology, *42:*379, 1948.

Schoenheimer, R.: Dynamic State of Body Constituents. Cambridge, Harvard University Press, 1946.

—— and Rittenberg, D.: Study of intermediary metabolism of animals with aid of isotopes. Physiol. Rev., *20:*218, 1940.

Selye, H.: Studies on adaptation. Endocrinology, *21:*169, 1937.

——: Textbook of Endocrinology. Montreal, Acta Endocrinologica, Université de Montreal, 1947.

Soffer, L. J., Gabrilove, J. L., and Jailer, J. W.: Role of adrenal in uptake of I^{131} by thyroid following parenteral administration of epinephrine. Proc. Soc. Exper. Biol. & Med., *71:*117, 1949.

——, Volterra, M., Gabrilore, L., Pollack, A., and Jacobs, M.: Effect of iodine and adrenalin on thyrotropin in Graves' disease and in normal and thyroidectomized dogs. Ibid., *64:*446, 1947.

Stevenson, J. A. F., Schenker, V., and Browne, J. S. L.: The 17-ketosteroid excretion in damage and convalescence. Endocrinology, *35:*216, 1944.

Talbot, N. B., Saltzman, A. H., Wixom, R. L., and Wolfe, J. K.: The colorimetric assay of urinary corticosteroid-like substances. J. Biol. Chem., *160:*535, 1945.

Thorn, G. W., Forsham, P. H., Prunty, F. T. G., and Hills, A. G.: Test for adrenal cortical insufficiency; response to pituitary adrenocorticotrophic hormone. J.A.M.A., *137:*1005, 1948.

Uotila, U. U.: The regulation of thyrotropic function by thyroxin after pituitary stalk section. Endocrinology, *26:*129, 1940.

Valentine, W. N., Craddock, C. G., Jr., and Lawrence, J. S.: Relation of adrenal cortical hormone to lymphoid tissue and lymphocytes. Blood, 3:729, 1948.
Venning, E., and Browne, J. S. L.: Excretion of glycogenic corticoids and of 17-ketosteroids in various endocrine and other disorders. J. Clin. Endocrinol., 7:79, 1947.
———, Kazmin, V. E., and Bell, J. C.: Biological assay of adrenal corticoids. Endocrinology, 38:79, 1946.
Vogt, M.: Output of cortical hormone by mammalian suprarenal. J. Physiol., 102:341, 1943.
———: Observations on some conditions affecting the rate of hormone output by the suprarenal cortex. Ibid., 103:317, 1944.
———: Biological assays of cortical hormones and estimation of rate of secretion of mammalian suprarenal cortex. J. Endocrinol., 5:lvii, 1947.
———: Cortical lipids of the normal and denervated suprarenal gland under conditions of stress. J. Physiol., 106:394, 1947.
White, A., and Dougherty, T. F.: Role of adrenal cortex and thyroid in mobilization of nitrogen from tissues in fasting. Endocrinology, 41:230, 1947.
Williams, R. H., Jaffe, H., and Kemp, C.: Effect of severe stresss upon thyroid function. Am. J. Physiol., 159:291, 1949.
Zaffaroni, A., Burton, B. R., and Keutmann, E. H.: Analysis of commercial adrenal cortex extracts by paper partition chromatography. Federation Proc., 9:250, 1950.

CHAPTER **2**

METABOLIC ASPECTS OF BODY FLUID REGULATION AND OF SHOCK

FLUID AND ELECTROLYTE METABOLISM

The regulation of body fluid and salt exchange is a very complex process. Moreover, the metabolism of these constituents is inextricably

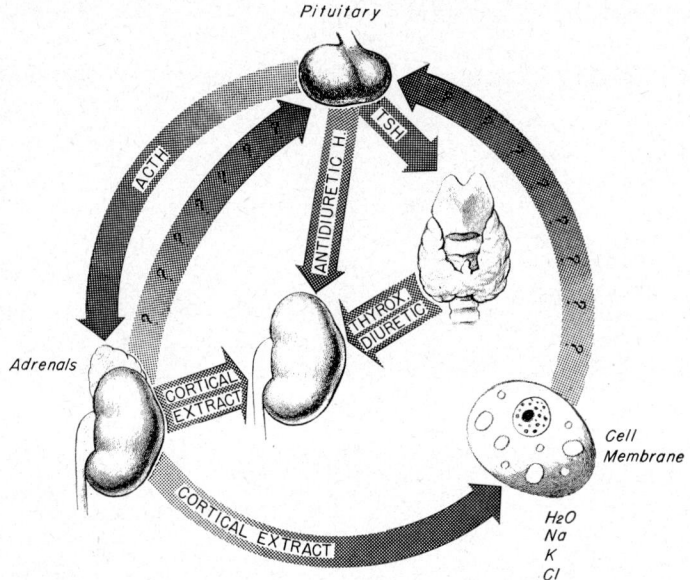

Endocrine Factors in Water and Salt Metabolism

Fig. 6. It has become crystal clear that endocrine influences play a major role in the maintenance of the normal volumes and composition of the body fluid compartments. Certain of these influences are indicated in the diagram and others are discussed in the text. ("Cortical extract" refers here to cortical hormones.)

linked with many other phases of metabolism. To cite a single example, a derangement in carbohydrate metabolism, as in diabetes mellitus, will profoundly influence the composition of virtually all body fluids. Clearly, a comprehensive consideration of the physiology of body water and electrolytes must not overlook these broader relationships. Nevertheless, some endocrine organs play an especially prominent role in the regulation of salt and water exchanges, and it is certain of these relationships which will be examined here. The endocrine organs which play a particularly important part in the regulation of the volume and composition of body fluid compartments are the two lobes of the pituitary, the adrenal cortex and the thyroid gland.

The Action of the Pituitary

The Anterior Lobe. The secretion of this lobe acts in at least two ways to affect the composition of body fluids. The first of these actions is mediated through the steroids of the adrenal cortex by means of the liberation of ACTH. The second mode of action is diuretic in nature and this effect is mediated through the secretion of TSH, which stimulates the thyroid to produce thyroxine with its well known diuretic properties. However, while the pituitary gland exercises a prominent and perhaps dominant regulatory action on the rates of secretion of both the thyroid and the adrenal, these target organs have a certain basic secretory rhythm which appears to be independent of pituitary stimulation (Sayers).

The Posterior Lobe. This lobe secretes the antidiuretic principle which acts on the renal tubules to increase water reabsorption. This hormone is secreted at a variable rate and its regulatory mechanism is sensitively responsive to varying states of hydration (Gaunt, Birnie and Eversole). Failure of the liver to inactivate the antidiuretic hormone at a normal rate, as in the chronic hepatic failure of cirrhosis, may result in the retention of excessive deposits of water which are manifested as edema and ascites (Ralli).

The Action of the Thyroid

The thyroid secretion, thyroxine, has a marked diuretic effect in the myxedematous patient and, to a lesser extent, in the euthyroid subject. While the precise role of the thyroid in diabetes insipidus is not clear, Keller found it exceedingly difficult if not impossible to produce permanent diabetes insipidus in experimental animals in the absence of the thyroid gland. The function of thyroxine in the fluid metabolism of the normal patient awaits further study.

The Action of the Adrenal Cortex

Under the stimulus of ACTH the adrenal cortex secretes numerous steroids which act in three general ways (Gaunt, Birnie and Eversole): First, there is a direct action on renal mechanisms, essentially independent of electrolyte metabolism, the effect of which is to regulate the rate and extent of water excretion. Second, cortical hormones cause sodium retention by the kidney, the osmotic consequence of which is a retention of water. Increased or decreased diuresis may result from the interaction of these two factors, depending upon the physiologic conditions at the time. Third, there are vaguely defined extrarenal processes by which the cortical hormones affect internal fluid distribution. Such factors involve the permeability of phase membranes. Most of the cortical substances studied have a diuretic influence, despite their variable effects on salt retention, but cortisone is a more effective diuretic than desoxycorticosterone. The substances most effective in inducing diuresis are least effective in causing salt retention.

The effects of the adrenal steroids on internal fluid distribution, as reflected in the size and composition of the body fluid compartments

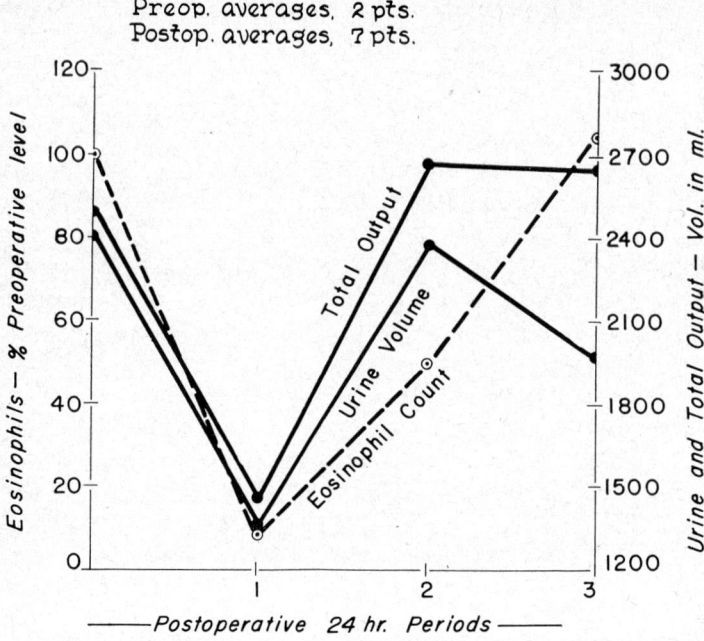

Fig. 7. Averages of output volumes and total eosinophil counts preoperatively and during the first three days postoperatively. Note the similarity of the three curves. The urinary volume and total output (urine plus gastrointestinal suction) are lowest when adrenocortical activity is maximal, as indicated by the profound fall in circulating eosinophils. (Hardy, J. D.: Ann. Surg., 132:189, 1950; J. B. Lippincott Company.)

(extracellular and intracellular) may emerge as being as important as the effects of these steroids on renal tubular function. Gaudino and Levitt, using the radioisotopes of sodium and potassium in conjunction with deuterium oxide (heavy water) for the measurement of body water, found that the administration of desoxycorticosterone in dogs caused a decrease in intracellular fluid volume, an increase in extracellular volume, and an increase in the intracellular concentrations of sodium and potassium. The administration of adrenocortical extract, on the other hand, increased the intracellular fluid volume. These workers found that there was a marked tendency to maintain a normal plasma volume. While these excellent studies need not be taken as the final word, they do indicate the remarkably specific effects which various of the C-21 adrenocortical steroids have on the transfer of water and electrolytes across the cell membrane. Additional support is derived from the finding of Overman that these hormones markedly affect the rates of radiosodium distribution in different body tissues.

Apparently, then, adrenocortical insufficiency results in an increase in the intracellular fluid volume, a decrease in the extracellular fluid volume, a decline in the serum sodium and chloride concentrations, and an increase in the serum level of potassium. Desoxycorticosterone reverses these relationships and actively promotes the renal excretion of potassium, presumably to some extent from the cells. However, in at least one respect the salt regulating activity of adrenocortical extract is not adequately replaced by desoxycorticosterone. Cortical extract maintains homeostasis of sodium in states of dietary excess as well as in dietary deficiency of this ion, while desoxycorticosterone induces renal retention of sodium regardless of intake.

The "amorphous fraction" which remains behind (with its striking effect on fluid and mineral metabolism) when all known adrenocortical steroids have been identified cannot be measured quantitatively, but Conn has used the analysis of sweat electrolytes before and following surgery to estimate the nature and duration of the changes effected by such "mineralo-corticoids." He has found that following major operations the sodium and chloride excretion in sweat decreases while the potassium content increases, as compared with the preoperative findings. These alterations may persist for a number of days before returning to normal levels. This same type of electrolytic pattern is reflected in the urine of such patients immediately following operation, though here the extent and duration of the changes are less striking. This same type of response is seen following the administration of ACTH or desoxycorticosterone. Such analyses of sweat may yield information that will be useful clinically.

CHANGES IN FLUID AND ELECTROLYTE METABOLISM FOLLOWING MAJOR SURGICAL PROCEDURES

Patients frequently present an oliguria in the immediate postoperative period. This low urinary volume is usually not the result of dehydration, effects of the anesthetic agent per se, or of a diminished circulating blood volume with incipient shock (Cooper, Iob and Coller). Rather, this temporary urinary suppression is probably the result of an increased activity of the adrenal cortex in response to the trauma of anesthesia and operation (Hardy; Johnson, Conn, Iob, and Coller). During this period of low urinary volume, the rate of urinary excretion of sodium and chloride is diminished but the rate of excretion of potassium is increased. Paralleling these changes in the urinary electrolytes, the blood analyses may show a physiologic hypochloremia, hyponatremia and, less com-

METABOLIC ASPECTS OF BODY FLUID REGULATION

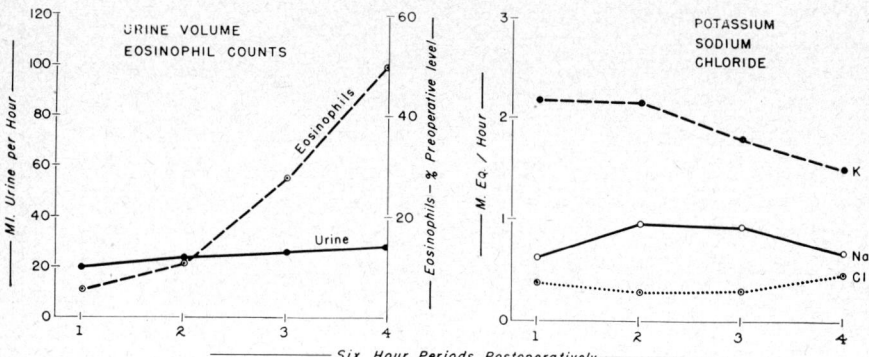

Fig. 8. Average rates of urinary excretion of water, potassium, sodium and chloride in the first four six-hour periods postoperatively. Observe the correlation with the total eosinophil counts. The rate of potassium excretion is increased immediately after operation, but this begins to subside after twelve to eighteen hours. (Hardy, J. D.: Ann. Surg., *132*:189, 1950; J. B. Lippincott Company.)

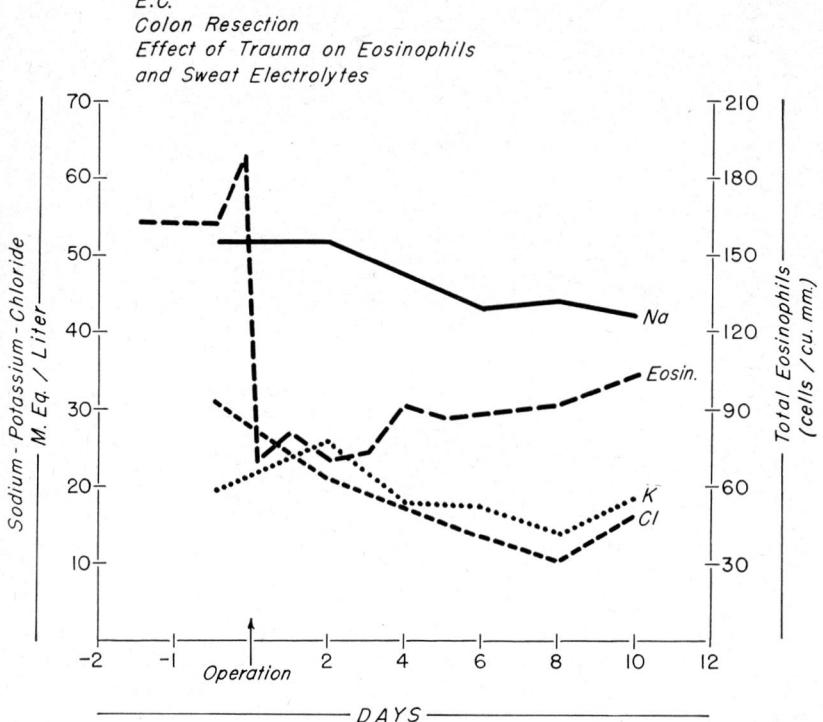

Fig. 9. Sweat was collected before and on every second day following operation, and its electrolyte composition was determined. In the immediate postoperative period the concentration of potassium was increased while that of sodium and chloride was decreased. These changes are characteristic of the alterations in the composition of sweat which follow trauma. Total eosinophil counts are presented to indicate variations in the level of adrenocortical activity.

monly, a hypokalemia. Since the loss of these ions from the body frequently has been quite small, these "low" blood levels of sodium, chloride and potassium may merely reflect a transfer of water from the intracellular to the extracellular fluid compartment, resulting in an increased absolute volume of the latter with a consequent dilution of the ions contained therein. Therefore, unless and until such electrolytic changes are proved harmful to the organism, it would seem prudent to regard them as purposeful shifts in the total response of the organism to stress. If

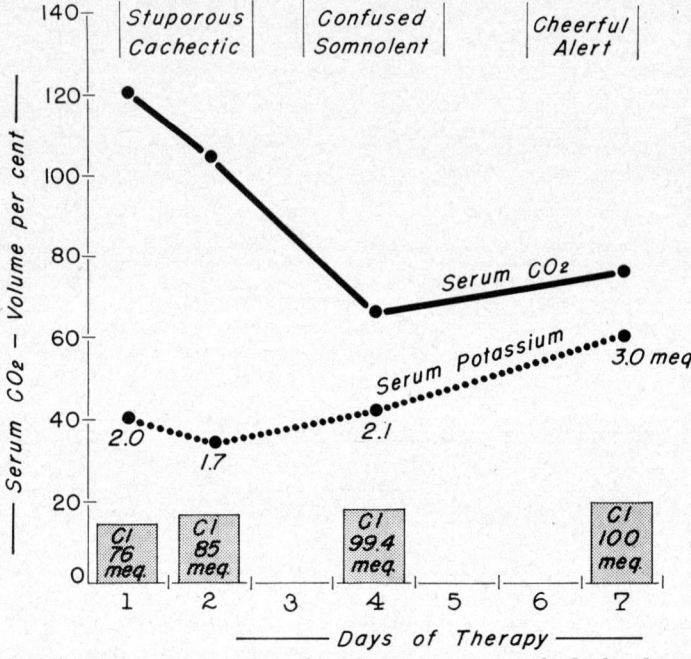

Fig. 10. Effects of reparative electrolyte therapy in a severely depleted patient. The electrolyte solutions used were potassium chloride (0.6 per cent potassium chloride in 0.45 per cent sodium chloride), ammonium chloride (2 per cent), and sodium chloride (0.85 per cent). Frequent determinations of the blood chemistry were employed to regulate rates of replacement. There exists at present no magic formula by which a patient's precise requirements can be calculated. (Hardy, J. D.: Pennsylvania M. J., 54:869, 1951.)

one views these phenomena from such a standpoint, it follows that it may be more logical to refrain from trying with replacement therapy to bring these serum electrolyte values to normal concentrations in the immediate postoperative period, if these changes are of only moderate degree.

The volume of intestinal fluid which can be aspirated with an indwelling tube and continuous suction is also diminished in the immediate postoperative period, and this finding also has been shown to bear an inverse relationship to changes in adrenocortical activity (Hardy). This finding has clinical importance. The abdominal surgeon is frequently dismayed

METABOLIC ASPECTS OF BODY FLUID REGULATION

when, following a bowel resection, the Miller-Abbott tube fails to drain what he considers an adequate volume. However, there need be no cause for concern when this drainage is small, so long as the abdomen remains soft and flat and the patient has no pain.

General Suggestions for Replacement Therapy in the Immediate Postoperative Period

1. The patient excretes much less sodium and chloride during the first 48 hours following operation than he did preoperatively. Since excessive fluid deposits are detrimental to the organism, only that sodium and chloride lost in the sweat and drainage from any source need be replaced. Keeping the patient "a bit on the dry side" is preferable to overhydration.

TABLE 3

CAUSES OF POSTOPERATIVE OLIGURIA AND HINTS CONCERNING THEIR MANAGEMENT

1. *Effects of increased adrenocortical activity on the renal tubules and on internal fluid distribution.* A normal response to trauma which will subside.
2. *Transfusion injury to the kidneys.* Recheck blood cross matching, examine urine for hemoglobin and red cells, and alkalinize patient immediately. Limit fluid intake to losses. Avoid "drowning" patient by maintaining his weight constant.
3. *Renal anoxia from poor respiratory exchange or prolonged hypotension during anesthesia.* The damage is often temporary and recovery under conservative management may usually be anticipated.
4. *Failure of chronically diseased kidneys to bear the added burden of anesthesia and operation.* The use of the artificial kidney may "rest" the patient's kidneys and permit recovery.
5. *Dehydration.* Administer appropriate fluids.
6. *Cardiac decompensation.* Employ digitalis and other measures as indicated.
7. *Hepatic failure.* A slow intravenous drip of 10 per cent glucose may be beneficial.
8. *Injuries to ureters, bladder, urethra, or renal blood supply at operation.* Nephrostomy, cystostomy, etc., as indicated.

2. The urinary volume is also diminished by physiologic mechanisms following major surgical procedures. There is no advantage in giving the patient several liters of fluid at a time when a total of only about two liters will be lost by sweat, urine, and vaporization in the lungs. Again, drainage should be replaced with electrolyte solutions.
3. A mild hypochloremia, hyponatremia and hypokalemia frequently result from "physiologic" fluid shifts between the intracellular and extracellular fluid compartments during the first twenty-four to forty-eight hours after operation. It is unlikely that any very useful purpose is served by attempting to correct minor variations in the concentrations of these ions. However, if persistent alkalosis attends a low serum potassium level, it is wise to administer this ion cautiously.
4. Deficits in fluids and electrolytes which could not be adequately

corrected preoperatively should continue to receive attention in the postoperative period.

THE RELATION OF ENDOCRINES TO ABNORMAL FLUID DEPOSITS

Ascites. There is a considerable body of evidence to support the view that, while a lowered serum protein level and an intrahepatic obstruction to the portal circulation play a significant role in the formation of

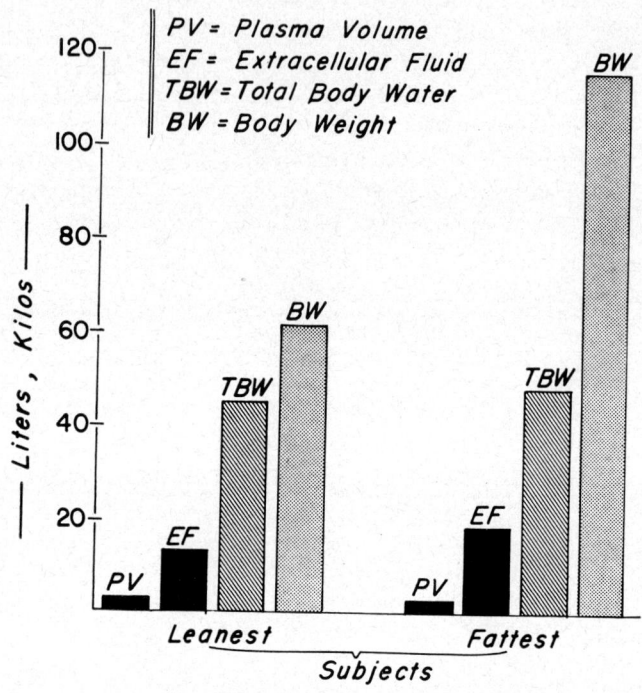

Fig. 11. Proportion of body fluid compartments to body fat in a very lean and in a very obese subject. While the obese subject weighed approximately twice as much as the lean subject, his total body water was only four liters greater. The thiocyanate space of the most obese subject was 18.2 liters, representing 37.6 per cent of the total body water and 15.7 per cent of the body weight. In contrast, the thiocyanate space of the leanest subject was 13.9 liters, representing 31.1 per cent of the total body water and 22.8 per cent of the body weight. The plasma volumes of these two individuals of approximately the same height but of markedly different weight and habitus were almost identical, being 3400 cc. and 3200 cc. (Hardy, J. D., Sen, P. K., and Drabkin, D. L.: Surg., Gynec. & Obst. 93:103, 1951; by permission of *Surgery, Gynecology and Obstetrics.*)

ascites, a diminished rate of inactivation of the antidiuretic hormone of the posterior pituitary is also an important contributing factor. Ralli and her associates have demonstrated that the urine of patients with cirrhosis increases antidiuretic activity when injected into hydrated rats. These investigators have drawn attention to the widely recognized fact that ascites may be absent in the presence of a markedly diminished serum protein level. Butt, Shell and Keys noted that patients with obstructive jaundice may have serum protein and oncotic pressure levels quite as low as those seen in cirrhotic patients, but that not nearly so many of the former develop ascites. The reduced urinary output of patients with ascites has long been recognized, and with a diet suitable for liver regeneration the cirrhotic patient may lose his ascites before the serum protein level has changed. An endocrine influence on the renal tubular excretion of sodium and chloride in cirrhosis has not been excluded.

Myxedema. This state of marked thyroid deficiency is particularly characterized by an edema-like appearance of the skin. However, this appearance is somewhat misleading. It is not a true edema but rather a deposit of a semifluid albuminous substance containing over 13 per cent protein (Means). This deposit is looked upon by Boothby and his associates as an increase in the normal quantity of stored or deposit protein. When thyroxine is administered, these patients excrete consid-

TABLE 4

THREE FACTORS IN ASCITES

1. Increased pressure in the portal system.
2. Decreased serum protein concentration (albumin especially important).
3. Diminished rate of inactivation of the pituitary antidiuretic hormone by the liver.

erable quantities of water and nitrogen. Thus, thyroxine is not only a diuretic, it is also an active agent in nitrogen mobilization.

Effects of Estrogens and Androgens. That estrogens may cause a retention of fluid has been observed for many years in connection with menstruation. The salt- and water-retaining effects of both estrogens and androgens have attained special clinical significance recently as a result of the widespread use of these agents in the palliative therapy of certain forms of advanced malignancy. Often the patient must be denied this type of relief for fear that the excessive fluid retention may precipitate pulmonary edema or cardiac failure. The mechanism by which these hormones cause this retention of fluid has not been established.

METABOLIC ASPECTS OF SHOCK

Shock has many faces. Despite the skills of generations of investigators, the fundamental physiologic failures which are reflected by the gross physical signs of shock that even the most casual observer can discern remain obscure. Nevertheless, this is not to imply that important advances have not been made. It is certain of these advances in our knowledge of metabolism in shock which we wish to present here.

Fairly early in the shock process the blood nitrogen rises because the destruction of liver enzymes results in a failure of this organ to remove amino acids from the blood stream. The degree of this rise in blood nitrogen has been used as a measure of the severity of hemorrhagic shock in experimental animals (Wilhelmi). Carbohydrate metabolism in the liver is also seriously impaired in shock. Rats in tourniquet shock fail to store glycogen in either the liver or muscles after the administration of glucose by tube. Insulin is not effective in causing glycogen storage under these circumstances, though there is a fall in blood sugar from the high levels characteristic of the early stages of tourniquet shock (Haist).

The brain and heart muscle maintain their energy reserves in relatively good order until shock is far advanced, and this may explain why many patients remain alert and attentive until a severe state of shock has intervened. Clearly the metabolic pattern of shock, as we now know it, is at least consistent with the view that the tissues are subjected to a progressively more severe anoxia owing to a prolonged reduction in blood oxygen supply. Moreover, the liver, the center of a surprisingly large segment of the metabolic activity of the body, emerges as a truly vital organ.

With this brief background, let us consider the evidence which supports the thesis that the liver is the organ primarily concerned with the prevention of "irreversible shock." Seligman, Frank and Fine, in a delightfully direct experiment, demonstrated in cross transfusion studies in dogs that if the liver of the shocked animal were continuously perfused with oxygenated blood from a donor dog, very severe grades of shock remained reversible. Concurrently Shorr, Zweifach and Furchgott developed experimental evidence to support their theory that the liver and the kidneys were chiefly implicated in the development of states of irreversible shock. They postulated that early in shock the kidneys produced a vaso-excitatory material (VEM) which enhanced the effect of epinephrine on the metarterioles and precapillaries. They showed that the kidney produced VEM both in vivo and in vitro, in the presence of anoxia. Both the kidney and the liver could destroy VEM anaerobically, but the capacity of the kidney to produce this material was lost after prolonged anoxia. In fact, as shock and anoxia deepened, VEM often disappeared from the blood stream. Meanwhile, the continued anoxia of the liver and muscles resulted in the production of a vasodepressor material (VDM) which depressed the response of the arterioles to epinephrine. These workers held that it was the function of the liver to destroy VDM quantitatively, though some of it might be excreted in the urine. A liver severely damaged by prolonged anoxia could no longer inactivate this material and, when this state has been reached, "irreversible shock" was at hand.

This theory fits in with many changes long recognized in shock, among which are pooling of the blood in the splanchnic vessels, passive edema, congestion and hemorrhage in the intestinal mucosa, increased intrahepatic resistance to blood flow with an increased portal pressure, apparent reduction of resistance in mesenteric vessels, and the trapping of red cells. Moreover, the concepts of Shorr and his associates are supported by many of the alterations in intermediary metabolism observed in shock, and their findings fit in with the transfusion experiments of Seligman and his associates.

It is of course too early to gain a balanced perspective of the light in which these investigations will ultimately be regarded, but it is not too early to recognize that these studies represent significant contributions to our understanding of an exceedingly complex process.

REFERENCES

Ariel, I., Kremen, A. J., and Wangensteen, O. H.: An expanded interstitial (thiocyanate) space in surgical patients. Surgery, 27:827, 1950.

Behnke, A. R.: Physiologic studies pertaining to deep sea diving and aviation, especially in relation to the fat content and composition of the human body (Harvey Lecture). Bull. New York Acad. Med., 18:561, 1942; Harvey Lect., 37:198, 1941–42.

Berliner, R. W.: Renal excretion of water and electrolytes. Amer. J. Med., 9:541, 1950.

Birnie, J. H., Eversole, W. J., Boss, W. R., Osborn, C. M., and Gaunt, R.: An antidiuretic substance in the blood of normal and adrenalectomized rats. Endocrinology, 47:1, 1950.

Boothby, W. M., Sandiford, I., Sandiford, K., and Slosse, J.: The effect of thyroxin on the respiratory and nitrogenous metabolism of normal and myxedematous subjects. I. A method of studying the reserve or deposit protein with a preliminary report of the results obtained. Tr. A. Am. Physicians, 40:195, 1925.

Butt, H. R., Snell, A. M., and Keys, A.: Plasma protein in hepatic disease: A study of colloid osmotic pressure of blood serum and the ascitic fluid in various diseases of the liver. Arch. Int. Med., 63:143, 1939.

Coller, F. A., Campbell, K. N., Vaughan, H. H., Iob, L. V., and Moyer, C. A.: Postoperative salt intolerance. Ann. Surg., 119:533, 1944.

Conn, J. W.: Electrolyte composition of sweat. Arch. Int. Med., 83:416, 1949.

——— and Louis, L. H.: Production of endogenous "salt-active" corticoids as reflected in the concentrations of sodium and chloride of thermal sweat. J. Clin. Endocrinol., 10:12, 1950.

Cooper, D. R., Iob, L. V., and Coller, F. A.: Response to parenteral glucose of normal kidneys and of kidneys of postoperative patients. Ann. Surg., 129:1, 1949.

Darrow, D. C.: Changes in muscle composition in alkalosis. J. Clin. Investigation, 25:324, 1946.

———, Pratt, E. L., Fleet, J., Jr., Gamble, A. H., and Wiese, H. F.: Disturbances of water and electrolytes in infantile diarrhea. Pediatrics, 3:129, 1949.

Fine, J., Seligman, A. M., and Frank, H. A.: Specific role of liver in hemorrhagic shock; report of progress to date. Ann. Surg., 126:1002, 1947.

Gaudino, M., and Levitt, M. F.: Adrenal cortex, body water and renal function. J. Clin. Investigation, 28:1487, 1949.

Gaunt, R., Birnie, J. H., and Eversole, W. J.: Adrenal cortex and water metabolism. Physiol. Rev., 29:281, 1949.

Haist, R. A.: Carbohydrate metabolism in traumatic shock. Am. J. Digest. Dis., 13:152, 1946.

Hardy, J. D.: The adrenal cortex and postoperative gastrointestinal secretions. Surgery, 29:517, 1951.

———: The role of the adrenal cortex in the postoperative retention of salt and water. Ann. Surg., 132:189, 1950.

——— and Drabkin, D. L.: The D_2O dilution space as a measure of total body water and the relation of body water to body size. Am. J. M. Sc., 219:108, 1949.

———, Sen, P. K., and Drabkin, D. L.: The relation of body fluid compartments to body fat and to each other. Surg., Gynec. & Obst., 93:103, 1951.

Heller, H., and Urban, F. F.: The fate of antidiuretic principle of post-pituitary extracts. J. Physiol., 85:502, 1935.

Hevesy, G., and Jacobson, C. F.: Rate of passage of water through capillary and cell walls. Acta physiol. scandinav., 1:11, 1940.

Ingle, D. J., Sheppard, R., Oberle, E. A., and Kuizenga, M. H.: A comparison of the acute effects of corticosterone and 17-hydroxycorticosterone on body weight and the urinary excretion of sodium, chloride, potassium, nitrogen and glucose in normal rat. Endocrinology, *39:*52, 1946.

Johnson H. T., Conn, J. W., Iob, V., and Coller, F. A.: Postoperative salt retention and its relation to increased adrenocortical function. Ann. Surg., *132:*374, 1950.

Keller, A. D.: Hypophyseal thyrotropic mechanism essential for occurrence of diabetes insipidus in its maximal form. Proc. Soc. Exper. Biol. & Med., *36:*787, 1937.

Labby, D., and Hoagland, C. L.: Water storage and the movements of body fluids and and chlorides during acute liver disease. J. Clin. Investigation, *26:*343, 1947.

Leslie, S. H., and Ralli, E. P.: The effect, in rats, of high fat diets on the renal excretion of water and antidiuretic substances. Endocrinology, *41:*1 1947.

McCance, R. A., and Widdowson, E. M.: A method for breaking down the body weights of living persons into terms of extracellular fluid, cell mass and fat and some applications of it to physiology and medicine. Proc. Roy. Soc., *138:*115, 1951.

Means, J. H.: The Thyroid and Its Diseases. 2d ed. Philadelphia, J. B. Lippincott Company, 1948.

Moore, F. D.: Determination of total body water and solids with isotopes. Science, *104:*157, 1946.

Moyer, C. A.: Acute temporary changes in renal function associated with major surgical procedures. Surgery, *27:*198, 1950.

———: Fluid and electrolyte balance. Surg., Gynec. & Obst., *84:*586, 1947.

Muntwyler, E., Griffin, G. E., Samuelsen, G. S., and Griffith, L. G.: The relation of the electrolytic composition of plasma and skeletal muscle. J. Biol. Chem., *185:*525, 1950.

Overman, R. R., Davis, A. K., and Bass, A. C.: Effect of cortisone and DCA on Na^{24} transport in adrenalectomized dogs. Federation Proc., *10:*100, 1951.

Ralli, E. P., Robson, J. S., Clarke, D., and Hoaglund, C. L.: Factors influencing ascites in patients with cirrhosis of the liver. J. Clin. Investigaton, *24:*316, 1945.

Sayers, G.: The adrenal cortex and homeostasis. Physiol. Rev., *30:*241, 1950.

——— and Sayers, M. A.: The pituitary-adrenal system. Recent Progr. Hormone Research, *2:*81, 1948.

Seligman, A. M., Frank, H. A., and Fine, J.: Traumatic shock: hemodynamic effects of alterations of blood viscosity in normal dogs and in dogs in shock. J. Clin. Investigation, *25:*1, 1946.

———, Frank, H. A., and Fine, J.: Traumatic shock; successful treatment of hemorrhagic shock by viviperfusion of liver in dogs irreversible to transfusion. Ibid., *26:*530, 1947.

Selye, H.: General adaptation syndrome and diseases of adaptation. J. Clin. Endocrinol., *6:*117, 1946.

Shorr, E., Zweifach, D. W., and Furchgott, R. F.: On occurrence, sites and modes of origin and destruction, of principles affecting compensatory vascular mechanisms in experimental shock. Science, *102:*489, 1945.

Soffer, L. J., Lesnick, G., Sorkin, S. Z., Sobotka, H., and Jacobs, M.: The utilization of intravenously injected salt in normals and in patients with Cushing's syndrome before and after administration of desoxycorticosterone acetate. J. Clin. Investigation, *23:*51 1944.

Thorn, G. W., Engel, L. L., and Lewis, R. A.: The effect of 17-hydroxycorticosterone and related adrenal cortical steroids on sodium and chloride excretion. Science, *94:*348, 1941.

———, Forsham, P. H., Prunty, F. T. G., and Hills, A. G.: Test for adrenal cortical insufficiency; response to pituitary adrenocorticotropic hormone. J.A.M.A., *137:*1005, 1948.

Waterhouse, C., and Keutmann, E. H.: Kidney function in adrenal insufficiency. J. Clin. Investigation, *27:*372, 1948.

Wilhelmi, A. E.: Metabolic aspects of shock. Ann. Rev. Physiol., *10:*259, 1947.

Zierler, K. L., and Lilienthal, J. L., Jr.: Sodium loss in man induced by desoxycorticosterone acetate: study in subject with myotonic dystrophy. Am. J. Med., *4:*186, 1948.

CHAPTER 3

THE DYNAMICS OF NUTRITION: THE RELATION OF NUTRITION TO AN ADEQUATE RESPONSE TO TRAUMA

The healing properties of food have been appreciated for centuries, and surgeons have recognized for a great many years that the starved patient is a poor operative risk. Until recently, however, the exact physiologic processes which are undermined by an inadequate diet were not known. Gradually the facts gathered from many isolated experiments are being integrated and certain incomplete pictures begin to emerge. A preliminary outline of selected aspects of protein, fat, carbohydrate and vitamin metabolism will be followed by a discussion of some specific effects of malnutrition on the alarm response.

PROTEIN METABOLISM IN STRESS CONDITIONS

"The primary function of protein foods is to supply the amino acids needed for the growth, repair, and general maintenance of the structural and catalytic machinery of living cells" (Baldwin).

The wealth of data on protein metabolism following trauma, particularly as reflected by the nitrogen balance, has been subjected to widely different analyses and interpretations. While the majority of students agree that there is usually a negative nitrogen balance following major operations, there exist at least three concepts as to why this occurs. The first is that of increased catabolism, supported particularly by the studies of Howard and of Cuthbertson, wherein there is an excessive breakdown of body tissue. The second is that of a failure of protein synthesis, "anti-anabolism," as discussed by Peters. The third, recently reaffirmed by Werner and his associates, postulates simply that in the immediate postoperative period the nutritional intake is inadequate and that nitrogen balance can be achieved by supplying the needed calories and protein. It appears not unreasonable at this time to preserve an open mind and to assume that under appropriate physiologic conditions any or all of these possibilities may obtain.

SPECIFIC ENDOCRINE EFFECTS ON NITROGEN METABOLISM

The increased nitrogen excretion which follows trauma has been considered by many to result from an increased activity of the adrenal cortex. Studies with ACTH and cortisone have usually shown a negative nitrogen balance following the administration of these compounds, an effect which, incidentally, can be reversed or prevented by the simultaneous administration of testosterone (Sprague and Power). Nevertheless, an increased adrenocortical activity is not the only cause of the negative nitrogen balance observed following trauma. Adrenalectomized

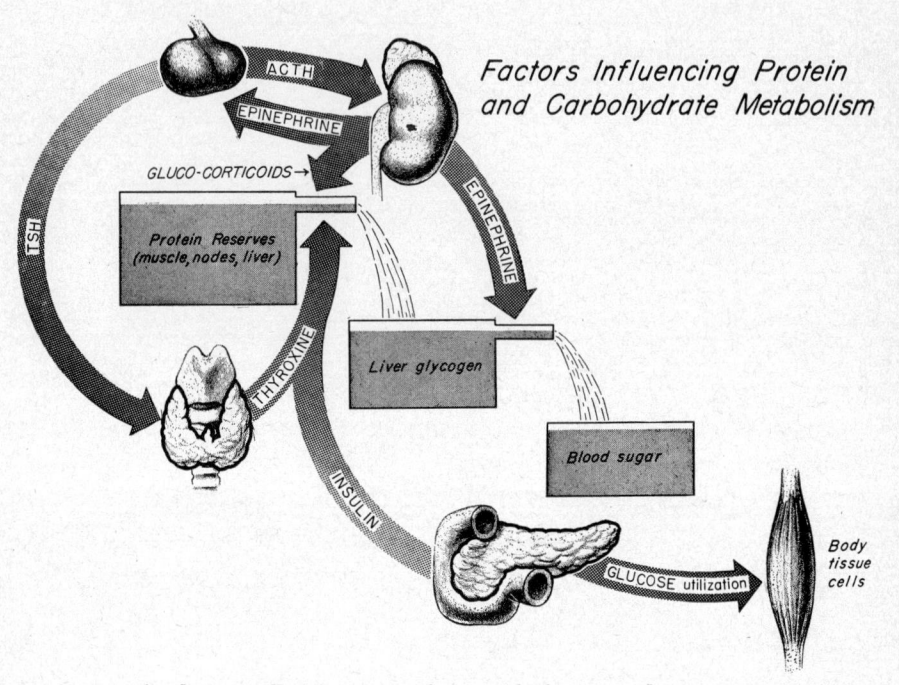

Fig. 12. The diagram illustrates some factors which may under appropriate physiologic conditions influence protein and carbohydrate metabolism. In stress an immediate but transient supply of carbohydrate fuel is supplied through the ability of epinephrine to promote the conversion of liver glycogen to glucose. If necessary, the glycogen reserves may then be replenished through the conversion of mobilized protein, a process in which the glucocorticoids of the adrenal cortex assume a prominent role. The action of insulin in liver glycogen formation and in glucose utilization is indicated. Thyroxine may have an important function in the mobilization of protein. (After Selye.)

animals maintained on a constant dose of adrenocortical extract still present an increased nitrogen output following trauma (Ingle). This finding has been extended by White and Dougherty, who have differentiated between the actions of the thyroid and the adrenals on nitrogen metabolism. Using starvation stress in mice, these workers found that the adrenal cortex had little effect in mobilizing nitrogen from the muscles. Thyroxine, on the other hand, mobilized nitrogen from the muscles but had little effect on the nitrogen of lymph nodes. However, these authors found that the presence of the adrenal cortical hormone was necessary for the thyroxine to exert its maximal effect. Neither thyroxine nor cortical extract was necessary for the partial mobilization of nitrogen from the

THE DYNAMICS OF NUTRITION

liver, but the presence of either substance could increase the amount of nitrogen mobilized from the liver. Their conclusion was that while a forty-eight hour fast in the normal mouse resulted in the loss of 31 per cent of the nitrogen of lymphoid tissues, 21 per cent of the nitrogen of the liver, and 12 per cent of the nitrogen of the carcass (muscle), the absolute amount of nitrogen lost from the carcass greatly outweighed that lost from the liver and lymph nodes. Thus, one is left with the inescapable implication that an altered level of thyroid activity may be of importance in the mobilization of nitrogen following surgical trauma.

FACTORS IN LIPID METABOLISM

Fats have at least two main functions: first, that of fuel reserves which are variable in amounts and, second, as an integral and constant part

Some Factors Influencing the Exchange of Lipids Between Fat Depots and the Liver

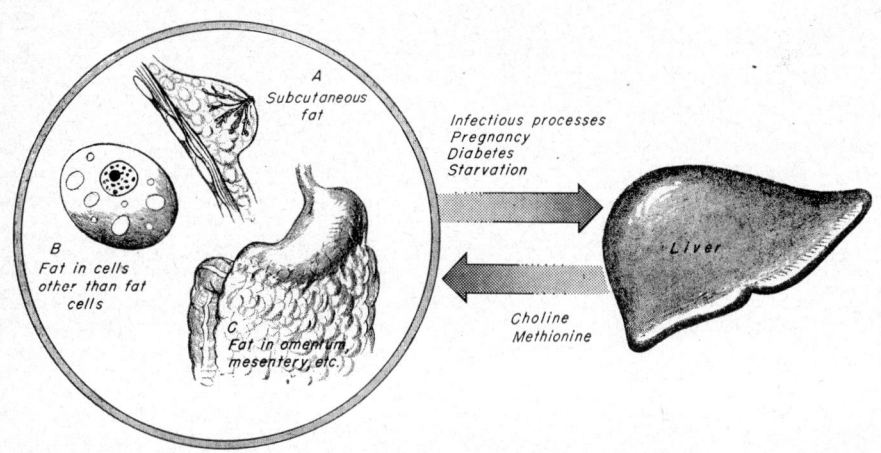

Fig. 13. In the diagram are represented several factors which influence the fat content of the liver. The fatty liver is more susceptible to injury by anoxia and certain anesthetic agents.

of the structure of living tissues. The rate of accretion of knowledge concerning the dynamics of lipid mobilization and transfer has lagged behind that concerning proteins and carbohydrates. Farmers had known for many years that the type of fat an animal deposited could be influenced by the diet he was fed when, in 1939, Schoenheimer and Rittenberg, using isotopic methods, demonstrated conclusively that there was a constant turnover of fatty acids in the body. Studies of this type have confirmed the view that the apparent constancy of the quantity of fat in the normal adult mammal results not from a chemical inertia of the fat depots but rather from the nice balance which exists between the processes leading to the deposition of fat and the processes leading to its mobilization and utilization. Furthermore, while the fatty acid composition of the fat deposited by farm animals can be altered by selective feeding, if permitted a wide dietary choice the animals will select those foods which form fat characteristic of the species.

The forces which mobilize fat from the depots and cause it to be transported to the liver, and the factors which increase the rate of turnover of fat in the liver with resulting storage in the depots, have come under critical scrutiny. The concept of *lipotropic* substances which either prevent the deposition of fat in the liver or accelerate its removal from this organ to the depots has been useful. Lipotropic factors include choline, methionine and inositol. They tend to prevent the accumulation of excess fat in the liver.

There are other powerful agents, *antilipotropic factors,* which increase fat deposition in the liver. The fatty liver seen in starvation stress has been shown by Best and Campbell to be due in part to the action of a factor derived from the anterior pituitary and endowed with the specific capacity of accelerating the mobilization of depot fat. Weil and Stettin have confirmed this finding and have suggested the name *adipokinin* for this material which they found excreted in the urine.

The thyroid gland has also been implicated as a controlling agent in fat transfer, and the correlation between hypothyroidism and an increased serum cholesterol level is well known. Nevertheless, varying experimental conditions in published reports render it impossible to decide at the present time whether or not the thyroid effect on clearing cholesterol from the liver is due to an increased transport and distribution or an altered synthesis and utilization of lipid substances.

ENDOCRINE INFLUENCES IN CARBOHYDRATE METABOLISM

The delicately balanced relationships between the pituitary, adrenal cortex, adrenal medulla and pancreas in the regulation of carbohydrate metabolism in the liver, muscles and other body tissues are so generally appreciated that they require little elaboration here. The blood sugar rises immediately following trauma and this hyperglycemia is due chiefly to the liberation of epinephrine which promotes glycogenolysis. This increment of blood sugar is fairly large but is of limited duration. This is in keeping with the postulate that an increased amount of glucose is one of the first needs of the organism subjected to stress. In more chronic stress, the response of the pituitary-adrenal axis results in the secretion of increased amounts of the glucocorticoids which increase the formation of glycogen from protein, thus maintaining the hepatic reserves of this quickly available fuel. The function of insulin is to promote glucose utilization and to inhibit gluconeogenesis from nonsugar reserves. Accordingly, insulin antagonizes the action of the glucocorticoids in this respect.

As with many other phases of thyroxine activity, its exact function in glucose metabolism has not been settled. Selye has reported that thyroidectomized animals show an exceptionally high blood sugar level in the general adaptation syndrome, and he suggests that this may be the result of poor glucose utilization. The glycosuria observed in hyperthyroidism is considered to be due to a poor glucose tolerance since, as a rule, neither the fasting blood sugar nor the renal threshold are abnormal (Means). Johnston believes that if the liver glycogen stores are kept filled in thyrotoxic human beings carbohydrate is burned not only as well as in normal persons but perhaps even better.

VITAMIN-ENDOCRINE RELATIONSHIPS

The nature of the essentiality of vitamins has been the subject of fruitful research. The activities of vitamins, endocrines and cellular processes are closely integrated. For example, Banerjee and Ghosh have shown that

TABLE 5

Why Vitamins Are Vital

---

1. Thiamine is believed to function in the cell as a coenzyme in the enzymatic transformation of α-keto acids, such as pyruvic and α-ketoglutaric acids, in reactions involving decarboxylation, oxidation, condensation, carbon dioxide fixation and dismutation (Best and Taylor).
2. Nicotinic acid and riboflavin appear to be necessary for the formation of compounds which are primarily concerned with the transport of hydrogen (Best and Taylor).
3. Severe vitamin C deficiency in guinea pigs may be accompanied by a diminution of the pancreatic insulin content to one-fourth of its normal level. This may account for the deranged carbohydrate metabolism seen in scurvy (Banerjee and Ghosh).
4. There appears to be a relationship between the level of vitamin A and thyroid activity (Means).
5. Vitamin D is essential for normal bone development.
6. Vitamin K is necessary for normal prothrombin formation.

---

in vitamin C deficiency in guinea pigs, the pancreatic insulin content may be lowered to one-fourth its normal level, resulting in a decreased glucose tolerance and a diminished liver glycogen content. These authors suggest that the disturbed carbohydrate metabolism seen in scurvy may be the result of insulin lack. In another approach to the relationship between insulin and vitamin C, Sherry and Ralli found that the injection of insulin caused a temporary decrease in the vitamin C content of plasma and urine. They concluded that this represented a transfer of the vitamin into the tissues, perhaps for some catalytic function. The administration of ACTH markedly decreases the normally high vitamin C content of the adrenal cortex (Sayers), but the exact significance of this practically constant finding has not been determined.

The role of thyroxine in promoting the conversion of carotene to vitamin A has been studied by Johnson and Baumann who found that, while the level of thyroid activity had no effect on the storage of preformed vitamin A in the liver and kidneys, the hyperthyroid animals fed carotene accumulated larger stores of vitamin A than did normal rats receiving equivalent amounts of carotene. Rats receiving thiouracil stored little vitamin A, but the subsequent administration of thyroxine to these same animals neutralized the effects of thiouracil and restored their ability to convert carotene to vitamin A. Moreover, increasing the basal metabolic rate with 2, 4-dinitrophenol did not increase the rate of conversion, indicating that thyroxine exerted a specific physiologic action in this respect.

The vital nature of the vitamins is further revealed by their close alliance with oxidative catalysts. Nicotinic acid is a constituent of certain nucleotides, and riboflavin enters into the structure of flavoproteins. Thus, these two vitamins appear to be necessary for the formation of compounds which are primarily concerned with the transport of hydrogen. Thiamine, in the form of thiamine pyrophosphate, is believed to function in the cell as a coenzyme in the enzymatic transformation of certain fatty acids. A relationship between thiamine and insulin is indicated by the observations of Foa, Smith and Weinstein that the increase in blood diphosphothiamine resulting from the intravenous injection of thiamine into dogs was considerably enhanced by a previous injection of insulin. Since the blood inorganic phosphorus also decreased slightly, the conclusion was reached that insulin catalyzed the phosphorylation of thiamine, possibly in the liver. In a different type of study, Deane and Shaw noted exhaustion effects in the zona fasciculata of the adrenal cortex of weanling rats in whom a severe dietary deficiency of thiamine had been produced. Finally, Axelrod and his associates have demonstrated a decreased antibody response in certain vitamin deficiencies.

From these selected observations it will be seen that the vitamins, in close association with hormones, affect such surgically important processes as the intermediary metabolism of carbohydrates, fats and proteins, antibody formation, tissue repair, hepatic function (including prothrombin formation) and the pituitary-adrenal response to stress.

SPECIFIC WAYS IN WHICH INADEQUATE NUTRITION REDUCES SURGICAL SUCCESS

That malnutrition and depleted states predispose to wound dehiscence, delayed function of anastomoses, delayed gastric empting time, decubitus ulcers and bacterial infections is widely recognized. These and other relationships are being clarified.

Nutrition and the Immediate Alarm Response

That the elements provided by an adequate preoperative dietary intake are needed at the very initiation of the response to stress has been shown in different ways. Forbes and associates demonstrated a diminished excretion of 17-ketosteroids in malnourished individuals following trauma, and these authors drew attention to the possible relationship between this diminished ketosteroid excretion and the lack of resistance of such patients to imposed stress. From a different approach, Moya and his coworkers found that a protein-rich regime augmented the ACTH response to stress. In the presence of a reduced adrenocortical secretion, it would seem reasonable to assume that the total metabolic activity of the individual may also be diminished.

We have seen that the myxedematous patient tolerates operation poorly. Many observers have pointed out the similarity between certain

TABLE 6

Effects of Malnutrition Which Decrease the Patient's Capacity to Withstand Trauma

Cardiovascular System
  1. Diminished blood volume
  2. Impaired circulatory reflexes
  3. Reduction in heart size
  4. Decreased cardiac output
  5. Increased sensitivity to drugs such as morphine
Fluid Metabolism
  1. Changes in cell membrane permeability
  2. Abnormal fluid deposits (edema, ascites) may interfere with wound healing, the functioning of gastrointestinal anastomoses and general metabolic activity.
Endocrine System
  1. Thyroid: The basal metabolism is diminished.
  2. Pituitary: Decreased output of ACTH in response to trauma.
  3. Adrenals: The urinary excretion of corticoids and 17-ketosteroids is diminished in severe malnutrition and the usual response to trauma is lacking.
  4. Pancreas: The insulin content of the pancreas may be markedly reduced in vitamin C deficiency.
Gastrointestinal System
  1. Intestinal digestion and absorption are defective in certain states of dietary deficiency.
Liver
  1. In starvation fat is mobilized from the depots and transported to the liver, increasing the vulnerability of this organ to anoxia and to certain anesthetic agents.
  2. Dietary deficiencies may in themselves result in marked liver damage.

features of hypothyroidism and starvation, and Husby has demonstrated a decrease in metabolism of nearly 5 per cent after only three to seven days on a low caloric diet.

The interdependence of thyroid and adrenal function in regulating cellular metabolic activity has been emphasized. Baldwin, in his discussion of the relationship between the hormones and an adequate dietary intake, draws attention to the close structural similarity between epinephrine and thyroxine on the one hand, and between phenylalanine and tyrosine on the other. He notes that insulin formation makes heavy demands on the supplies of essential amino acids and points out that at least a modicum of formation of such special products as hormones and enzymes must continue in starvation, even at the expense of tissue protein.

The immediate alarm response frequently involves a reaction to the invasion of bacteria, and it has been shown in animals that both vitamin and protein deficiencies decrease the antibody response. Balch has recently published data which conflict with such studies but it seems likely that marked deficiencies, with their detrimental effects on total cellular activity, do influence antibody formation unfavorably.

Nutrition and Hepatic Function

The liver occupies a commanding position in the preservation of body homeostasis under both normal conditions and in stress. The importance of the dietary intake in protecting this organ from damage by noxious agents and in permitting rapid regeneration has been recorded by numerous students in this field. As noted previously, Best and Campbell have shown that starvation per se results in a mobilization of the peripheral fat depots with a resulting lipemia and an increase in hepatic lipids. The poor toleration of the fatty liver for certain anesthetic agents has been amply demonstrated (Goldschmidt, Vars and Ravdin). A qualitative protein deficiency has been shown by Rao and others to result in an acute massive hepatic necrosis in animals. Those which survived the acute necrosis developed postnecrotic scarring and nodular hyperplasia. On the other hand, a diet adequate in protein but deficient in lipotropic factors, such as choline, resulted in a fatty infiltration of the liver which developed into a diffuse fibrosis. Entenman, Chaikoff and Reichert reported that the development of fatty livers previously reported in hypophysectomized-thyroidectomized dogs fed on a high protein diet could be prevented by the daily administration of two grams of free choline chloride. This agent failed, however, to prevent a rise in blood lipids. On the basis of such data, it was suggested that the effectiveness of lipotropic constituents of the normal diet depends upon the action of the thyroid hormone.

It has been seen that prolonged malnutrition may result in a failure of the liver effectively to neutralize the antidiuretic factor of the posterior pituitary. The ascites which may result can frequently be reversed by a high protein diet, this even before any change in the serum protein level is detected (Ralli).

Salter, Klatskin and Humm concluded that the gynecomastia prevalent among American troops in Japanese prison camps was a result of the failure of a liver depleted of proteins and vitamins efficiently to neutralize estrogens, while at the same time the liver retained its ability to neutralize androgens. In France, Lamy, Lamotte and Lamotte-Barrillon observed many signs of severe hypothyroidism as well as diminished function of other endocrine glands in camp internees.

Cardiovascular Reflexes and Plasma Volume

Taylor, Henschel and Keys studied cardiovascular dynamics in semistarved people and found, in addition to a diminished plasma volume, a poor tolerance for postural changes induced by the tilt table. These observers found no adequate explanation for this. They noted in some of these subjects a pitting edema which was associated with little or no fall in the serum protein level. Muscular strength and the ability to maintain a balanced emotional outlook were also impaired.

THE ADEQUATE DIET

Route of Administration. The most convenient and effective route for feeding surgical patients is by mouth. The evidence indicates that materials so introduced are more efficiently utilized than when administered intravenously. Moreover, it is seldom possible to achieve really adequate nutrition by the parenteral route.

The Appearance and Serving of the Diet. The patient appreciates warm food served attractively. The psychologic effect on the appetite of careful planning in this respect cannot be overemphasized. The very patients who are in the greatest need of nutritive restoration are apt to be the ones whose appetite is the most capricious.

Appetite. Contrary to previous opinion, the stomach is not the primary seat of the appetite. The evidence now indicates that there is a central mechanism for this symptom that is not dependent on sensory stimuli from the stomach and intestine. For instance, patients who have had a total gastrectomy do not lose their appetite. Ginsberg, Feldman and Necheles found that unpleasant odors which abolished the appetite in human beings did not stop hunger contractions in dogs and humans. Adolph showed that nonnutritive materials did not appease hunger or satisfy the appetite. The measurement of olfactory acuity has been suggested as a method for the quantitation of the appetite, since there appears to be a direct correlation between the sensitivity of the sense of smell and the intensity of the desire for food.

Vitamins. The minimum daily vitamin requirements have been detailed in numerous texts. In view of our increasing knowledge of the unique positions which these agents occupy in the cellular metabolic machinery, it would seem advisable to supply the patient with liberal amounts of all known vitamins.

Protein Administration. The desirability of overcoming the negative nitrogen balance which exists following operation has been questioned by some on the grounds that such nitrogen loss is "physiologic." However, the trauma which produced the nitrogen loss was not "physiologic," and it would seem appropriate to support the injured patient with a diet which at least equals what he would have consumed had he not been injured. We do not subscribe to the thesis that fasting does the patient no harm. Although there may be a brief period of either increased catabolism and/or anti-anabolism immediately following operation, the exact time relationships of these processes have not been defined and, even at the risk of "wasting" nutritive materials by introducing them at a time when they will not be utilized, it seems worthwhile to have the building materials available in anticipation of such a time as the body will be able to use them for fuel or for tissue fabrication.

The amount of protein and nonprotein calories required by the surgical patient has been the subject of many investigations. Unless basic caloric needs are met, the administered protein, or its tissue equivalent as needed, will be burned for fuel. Benditt and his associates suggest that the afebrile patient in bed without stimulants requires 1500 calories of

TABLE 7

SOLUTIONS WHICH MAY BE USED FOR INTRAVENOUS ALIMENTATION, WITH APPROXIMATE CALORIC VALUES

1. Glucose solution with or without saline
    - 5% glucose = 200 cal./liter
    - 10% glucose = 400 cal./liter
2. Protein hydrolysate
    - 5% amino acid mixture = 200 cal./liter
    - 5% glucose = 200 cal./liter
    - Total = 400 cal./liter
3. Protein hydrolysate with alcohol
    - 5% amino acid mixture = 200 cal./liter
    - 5% glucose = 200 cal./liter
    - 7% absolute alcohol (200 proof)
    - (70 cc. at approximately 7 cal./cc.) = 490 cal./liter
    - Total = 890 cal./liter

    N.B.: The alcoholic solution must be infused slowly to achieve sedation and alimentation while avoiding intoxication. We recommend that not more than two liters of this solution be administered during each twenty-four hour period. Three liters of protein hydrolysate make available to the patient 150 gm. of split protein derivatives.
4. Intravenous fat

    This work is still in the experimental stage, but the results thus far are most encouraging (Stare). Such a mixture would afford the patient nine calories for each gram of fat infused.

nonprotein energy per day if protein is not to be burned. In the presence of fever this value must be revised upward. Moreover, since the therapeutic goal is not the mere maintenance of nitrogen equilibrium but the fabrication of significant quantities of body protein, protein levels of the order of 2 to 4 gm. per kilogram of body weight per day are demanded for the rapid rehabilitation of the depleted man. At these levels there is both a higher gross efficiency of protein utilization and greater absolute protein gain. Riegel and her coworkers recommend at least 0.3 gm. of nitrogen and 30 calories per kilo each twenty-four hours. Again, in the presence of excessive needs such as occur in markedly febrile postoperative courses, these figures must be raised.

Caloric Intake. Carbohydrate has in the past been the most easily available substance for the intravenous administration of calories. Perhaps this was a happy circumstance since, as we have seen, glucose is one of the first needs of the organism in stress. However, intravenous fat yields over twice the number of calories as does carbohydrate. Stare has prepared a fat emulsion suitable for intravenous administration in human beings but, unfortunately, pyrogenic reactions have been frequent. Nevertheless, it now appears certain that such a preparation will

TABLE 8

Successful Gastrostomy Formulas, with Approximate Food and Caloric Values
(Formulas Devised by Miss Marie T. Wackerman, A.D.A.)

	PROTEIN grams	FAT grams	CARBOHYDRATE grams	CALORIES
1. Skimmed milk, 1000 cc. Whole milk, 1000 cc. Eggs, 2 Proteinum, 200 gm. Dextri-Maltose No. 2, 100 gm. Polyvitamin Dispersion, 2 tsp. Approximate values	162	62	287	2354
2. Casec, 200 gm. Skimmed milk, 2000 cc. Vegetable oil, 170 cc. Polyvitamin Dispersion, 2 tsp. Approximate values	240	186	96	3018
3. Skimmed milk, 2000 cc. Casec, 200 gm. Strained vegetables to 3000 cc. Polyvitamin Dispersion, 2 tsp. Approximate values	250	16	131	1668
4. Skimmed milk, 1500 cc. Alacta, 180 gm. Eggs, 9 Egg whites, 3 Sucrose, 450 gm. Salt, 8 gm. Approximate values	191	79	605	3895

N.B. Kaopectate may be added and homogenized milk may be substituted if the patient exhibits a tendency toward loose stools.

soon be available commercially and will fulfill the great remaining need in intravenous alimentation, namely, the introduction of abundant calories.

REFERENCES

Adolph, E. F.: Inability of non-nutritive materials to satisfy appetite (or appease hunger).. Am. J. Physiol., *151*:110, 1947.

Allison, J. B., Seeley, R. D., Brown, J. H., and Ferguson, F. P.: Effects of depletion and repletion in proteins on body fluids in adult dogs. Proc. Soc. Exper. Biol. & Med., *63*:214, 1946.

Axelrod, A. E., Carter, B. B., McCoy, R. H., and Geisinger, R.: Circulating antibodies in vitamin-deficiency states. Proc. Soc. Exper. Biol. & Med., *66*:137, 1947.

Balch, H. H.: Antibody formation in malnourished patients; in American College of

Surgeons: Surgical Forum (Proceedings of the Forum Sessions, Thirty-Sixth Clinical Congress of the American College of Surgeons). Philadelphia, W. B. Saunders Company, 1951, p. 466.

Baldwin, E.: Dynamic Aspects of Biochemistry. New York, The Macmillan Company, 1947.

Banerjee, S., and Ghosh, N. C.: Relation of scurvy to glucose tolerance test, liver glycogen, and insulin content of pancreas of guinea pigs. J. Biol. Chem., 168:207, 1947.

Barker, S. B.: Metabolic functions of the endocrine system. Ann. Rev. Physiol., 12: 45, 1949.

Benditt, E. P., Humphreys, E. M., Wissler, R. W., Steffee, C. H., Frazier, L. E., and Cannon, P. R.: Dynamics of protein metabolism. J. Lab. & Clin. Med., 33:257, 1948.

———, Woolbridge, R. L., and Stepto, R.: Protein dynamics; relationship between level of protein intake and rate of protein utilization by protein depleted men and rats. Ibid., 269.

Benedict, F. G., Miles, W. R., Roth, P., and Smith, H. M.: Human Vitality and Efficiency Under Prolonged Restricted Diet. (Carnegie Institute Publication No. 280.) Washington, The institute, 1919. (Quoted by Keys, et al., Human Starvation, vol. 1, p. 313.)

Best, C. H., and Campbell, J.: Anterior pituitary extracts and liver fat. J. Physiol., 86: 190, 1936.

——— and Taylor, N. B.: The Physiological Basis of Medical Practice, 4th ed. Baltimore, The Williams & Wilkins Company, 1945.

Browne, J. S. L., Schenker, V., and Johnson, L. G.: Urinary corticoid excretion studies in a patient with panhypopituitarism; in Transactions of the Fifteenth Conference on Metabolic Aspects of Convalescence. New York, Josiah Macy, Jr., Foundation, 1948, p. 154.

Carter, B. B., and Axelrod, A. E.: Circulating antibodies in vitamin deficiency states; thiamin and biotin deficiencies. Proc. Soc. Exper. Biol. & Med., 67:416, 1948.

Cuthbertson, D. P.: Observations on the disturbance of metabolism produced by injury to the limbs. Quart. J. Med., 1:233, 1932.

———, McGirr, J. L., and Robertson, J. M. S.: The effect of fracture of bone on the metabolism of the rat. Quart. J. Exper. Physiol., 29:13, 1939.

Deane, H. W., and Shaw, J. H.: A cytochemical study of the responses of the adrenal cortex of the rat to thiamine, riboflavin, and pyridoxine deficiencies. J. Nutrition, 34:1, 1947.

Engel, F. L.: Role of the adrenal cortex in intermediary metabolism. Am. J. Med., 10:556, 1951.

———: Studies on the nature of the protein catabolic response to adrenal cortical extract. Accentuation by insulin hypoglycemia. Endocrinology, 45:170, 1949.

——— and Engel, M. G.: Urea synthesis from amino acids during hemorrhagic shock in the nephrectomized rat. Am. J. Physiol., 147:165, 1946.

———, Schiller, S., and Pentz, E. I.: Studies on the nature of the protein catabolic response to adrenal cortical extract. Endocrinology, 44:458, 1949.

Entenman, C., Chaikoff, I. L., and Reichert, F. L.: Influence of hypophysectomy, thyroidectomy, and of both hypophysectomy and thyroidectomy upon fat content of liver of dogs. Endocrinol., 42:210, 1948.

Foa, P. P., Smith, J. A., and Weinstein, H. R.: Effect of insulin on concentration of diphosphothiamine in blood. Arch. Biochem., 13:449, 1947.

Forbes, A. P., Donaldson, E. C., Reifenstein, E. C., Jr., and Albright, F.: Effect of trauma and disease on urinary 17-ketosteroid excretion in man. J. Clin. Endocrinol., 7:264, 1947.

Gaston, E. A.: Total pancreatectomy. New England J. Med., 238:345, 1948.

Geyer, R. P., Mann, G. V., and Stare, F. J.: Parenteral nutrition. IV. Improved techniques for the preparation of fat emulsions for intravenous nutrition. J. Lab. & Clin. Med., 33:153, 1948.

Ginsberg, R. S., Feldman, M., and Necheles, H.: Effect of odors on appetite. Gastroenterology, 10:281, 1948.

Goldschmidt, S., Vars, H. M., and Ravdin, I. S.: Influence of foodstuffs upon susceptibility of liver to injury by chloroform, and probable mechanism of their action. J. Clin. Investigation, 18:277, 1939.

Handler, P. J.: Influence of thyroid activity on liver and plasma lipides of choline- and cystine-deficient rats. J. Biol. Chem., 173:295, 1948.

Homburger, F., Abels, J. C., and Young, N. F.: Observations on normal young woman given synthetic 11-dehydrocorticosterone acetate. Am. J. Med., 4:163, 1948.

Howard, J. E., Winternitz, J., Parson, W., Bigham, R. S., Jr., and Eisenberg, H.: Fracture convalescence; influence of diet on post-traumatic nitrogen deficit exhibited by patients. Bull. Johns Hopkins Hosp., 75:209, 1944.

Husby, J.: Decreases in metabolism averaging nearly five per cent after only three to seven days on a low caloric diet. Acta med. scandinav., 130:20, 1948.

Ingle, D. J.: Some studies on the role of the adrenal cortex in organic metabolism. Ann. New York Acad. Sci., 50:576, 1949.

Johnson, R. M., and Baumann, C. A.: The effect of thyroid on the conversion of carotene into vitamin A. J. Biol. Chem., 171:513, 1947.

Johnston, J. A.: Carbohydrate metabolism. II. Role of the thyroid gland. Am. J. Dis. Child., 48:1015, 1934.

Keys, A., Brozek, J., Henschel, A., Mickelsen, O., and Taylor, H. L.: The Biology of Human Starvation. 2 vols. Minneapolis, The University of Minnesota Press, 1950.

———, Taylor, H. L., Mickelsen, O., and Henschel, A.: Famine edema and mechanism of its formation. Science, 103:669, 1946.

Koelsche, G. A., and Kendall, E. C.: The relation of suprarenal cortical hormone to nitrogen metabolism in experimental hyperthyroidism. Am. J. Physiol., 113:335, 1935.

Lamy, M., Lamotte, M., and Lamotte-Barrillon, S.: Glandes endocrines et dénutrition. Ann. d'endocrinol., 8:437, 1947.

Landau, R. L., Knowlton, K., Anderson, D., Brandt, M. B., and Kenyon, A. T.: The effects of starvation on urinary 17-ketosteroid excretion. J. Clin. Endocrinol., 8:133, 1948.

Leblond, C. P., Gross, J., Peacock, W., and Evans, R. D.: Metabolism of radioiodine in the thyroids of rats exposed to high or low temperatures. Am. J. Physiol., 140:671, 1944.

Lehninger, A. L.: Role of metal ions in enzyme systems. Physiol. Rev., 30:393, 1950.

Long, C. N. H.: Conditions associated with secretion of adrenal cortex. Federation Proc., 6:46, 1947.

———: Factors regulating the adrenal cortical secretion; in American Association for the Advancement of Science, Section on Medical Sciences: Pituitary-Adrenal Function. Washington, The association, 1951, p. 24.

———, Katzin, B., and Fry, E.: The adrenal cortex and carbohydrate metabolism. Endocrinology, 26:309, 1940.

McKee, F. W., Schloerb, P. R., Schilling, J. A., Tishkoff, G. H., and Whipple, G. H.: Protein metabolism and exchange as influenced by constriction of vena cava; experimental ascites and internal plasmapheresis; sodium chloride and protein intake predominant factors. J. Exper. Med., 87:457, 1948.

Means, J. H.: The Thyroid and Its Diseases. 2d ed. Philadelphia, J. B. Lippincott Company, 1948.

Miller, E. V. O., Mickelsen, O., and Keys, A.: Urinary excretion of 17-ketosteroids by normal young men during starvation. Proc. Soc. Exp. Biol. & Med., 67:288, 1948.

Moya, F., Prado, J. L., Rodríguez, R., Savard, K., and Selye, H.: Effect of the dietary protein concentrations upon secretion of adrenocorticotrophin. Endocrinology, 42:223, 1948.

Nelson, R. A.: The pathophysiology of diabetes mellitus. Am. J. Digest. Dis., 14:352, 1947.

Perry, W. F., and Gemmell, J. P.: The effect of surgical operations on the excretion of iodine, corticosteroids, and uric acid. Canad. J. Research, 27:320, 1949.

Persike, E. C.: Increased protein catabolism in thyroidectomized rats; rates of urine urea excretion and serum urea concentrations. Endocrinology, 42:356, 1948.

Peters, J. P.: Problems of nitrogen metabolism. Federation Proc., 3:197, 1944.

——— and Man, E. B.: The interrelations of serum lipids in normal persons. J. Clin. Investigation, 22:707, 1943.

Price, W. H., Cori, C. F., and Colowick, S. P.: Effect of anterior pituitary extract and insulin on hexokinase reaction. J. Biol. Chem., *160*:133, 1945.
Ralli, E. P., Robson, J. S., Clarke, D., and Hoagland, C. L.: Factors influencing ascites in patients with cirrhosis of the liver. J. Clin. Investigation, *24*:316, 1945.
Rao, R.: Dietetic hepatic lesions and protein deficiency. Nature, *161*:446, 1948.
Ravdin, I. S., and Gimbel, N.: Protein metabolism in surgical patients. J.A.M.A., *144*: 979, 1950.
—— and Vars, H. M.: Further studies on factors influencing liver injury and liver repair. Ann. Surg., *132*:362, 1950.
Rawson, R. W. and McArthur, J. W.: Radioiodine: its use as a tool in the study of thyroid physiology. J. Clin. Endocrinol., *7*:235, 1947.
Reiss, M.: Lactogenic hormone and fat metabolism. Endocrinology, *40*,294, 1947.
Riegel, C., Koop, C. E., Drew, J., Stevens, L. W., and Rhoads, J. E.: The nutritional requirements for introgen balance in surgical patients during the early postoperative period. J. Clin. Investigation, *26*:18, 1947.
Risser, W. C., Olsen, R. T., Walther, O. H., and Doede, E. W.: Evaluation of proteins by the nitrogen balance method. J. Nutrition, *32*:485, 1946.
Rupp, J., and Paschkis, K. E.: Nitrogen sparing (protein-anabolic) action of thyroid hormone. J. Clin. Endocrinol., *8*:608, 1948.
Salter, W. T., Klatskin, G., and Humm, F. D.: Gynecomastia due to malnutrition. II. Endocrine studies. Am. J. M. Sc., *213*:31, 1947.
Sayers, G.: The adrenal cortex and homeostasis. Physiol. Rev., *30*:241, 1950.
—— and Sayers, M. A.: Pituitary-adrenal system. Recent Progr. Hormone Research, *2*:81, 1948.
Schoenheimer, R.: The Dynamic State of Body Constituents. Cambridge, Harvard University Press, 1946.
—— and Rittenberg, D.: Study of intermediary metabolism of animals with aid of isotopes. Physiol. Rev., *20*:218, 1940.
Selye, H.: Textbook of Endocrinology. Montreal, Acta Endocrinologica, Université de Montreal, 1947.
Sherry, S., and Ralli, E. P.: Further studies of effects of insulin on metabolism of vitamin C. J. Clin. Investigation, *29*:217, 1948.
Sprague, R. G., Gastineau, C. F., Mason, H. L., and Power, M. H.: Effects of synthetic 11-dehydrocorticosterone (compound A) in subject with Addison's disease. Am. J. Med., *4*:175, 1948.
——: Cortisone and ACTH: a review of certain physiologic effects and their clinical implications. Ibid., *10*:567, 1951.
—— and Power, M. H.: Metabolic effects of cortisone and ACTH; in American Association for the Advancement of Science, Section on Medical Sciences: Pituitary-Adrenal Function. Washington, The assocation, 1951, p. 132.
Stare, F. J., and Geyer, R. P.: Fat in parenteral nutrition. Surg., Gynec. & Obst., *92*: 246, 1951.
Stewart, J. D., Hale, H. W., Jr., and Schaer, S. M.: Management of protein deficiency in surgical patients, intravenous and intrajejunal injections. J.A.M.A., *136*:1017, 1948.
Taylor, H. L., Erickson, L., Henschel, A., and Keys, A.: The effects of bed rest on the blood volume of normal young men. Am. J. Physiol., *144*:227, 1945.
——, Henschel, A., and Keys, A.: Cardiovascular response to posture and the problem of faintness and syncope in the semi-starved individual. Ibid., *152*:141, 1948.
Thorn, G. W., Forsham, P. H., Frawley, T. F., Wilson, D. L., Renold, A. E., Fredrickson, D. S., and Jenkins, D.: Advances in the diagnosis and treatment of adrenal insufficiency. Am. J. Med., *10*:595, 1951.
Wang, C. F., Lapi, A., and Hegsted, D. M.: Studies on minimum protein requirements of adult dogs. J. Lab. & Clin. Med., *33*:462, 1948.
Weil, R., and Stetten, D., Jr.: The urinary excretion of a fat-mobilizing agent. J. Biol. Chem., *168*:129, 1947.
Werner, S. C.: Some effects upon nitrogen balance of the independent variation of proteins and calories in man. J. Clin. Investigation, *27*:561, 1948.

Werner, S. C.: Problems of parenteral nutrition. Am. J. Med., 5:749, 1948.
White, A., and Dougherty, T. F.: Role of adrenal cortex and thyroid in mobilization of nitrogen from tissues in fasting. Endocrinology, 41:230, 1947.
White, H. L., Heinbecker, P., and Rolf, D.: Endocrine influences on cardiac output and oxygen consumption in dogs. Am. J. Physiol., 151:239, 1947.
Wilder, J.: Anterior pituitary and pancreas. Am. J. Digest. Dis., 15:183, 1948.

CHAPTER 4

THE PHYSIOLOGIC BASIS OF EARLY AMBULATION: NOTES ON CONVALESCENCE

The physiologic basis of early ambulation is at the same time the physiology of convalescence, for the term convalescence embraces the return to normal of a multitude of metabolic activities in an individual who has sustained injury. These activities recover at different rates, and the recovery of many of them is not manifested by any objective and often no subjective sign. Quite simply, there eventually comes a time when the patient "feels well" and announces that he is ready to return to work. These changes which restore the patient to health are, for the most part, unknown.

Nevertheless, if early ambulation is to rest on a sound physiologic basis it must, at the very least, be demonstrated that the prompt mobilization of the surgical patient does not retard the overall return to health. Fortunately, a respectable body of evidence supports the view that early ambulation hastens the total rehabilitation of the individual following injury.

BACKGROUND OF EARLY AMBULATION IN THE UNITED STATES

As early as 1899 Emil Ries advocated the more prompt mobilization of patients following laparotomy, and in the ensuing years other sporadic voices were raised against the use of prolonged bed rest in medical as well as surgical diseases. Continental internists had never subscribed as completely to the dictum that prolonged bed rest was the first consideration in the treatment of all ills as had the surgeons. Particularly among European cardiologists was the patient permitted a degree of activity far exceeding that allowed in this country. In 1927 Harrison became convinced of the need for an entirely new evaluation of our use of bed rest as a primary means of therapy in heart disease, and his writings gave impetus to a movement whose beginnings could have been remarked several years sooner. Yet, it was not until the beginning of the fifth decade of this century that through the efforts of Leithauser, Powers and others surgical opinion was influenced in such a manner that ambulation of the patient on the day following even very serious operations became a routine practice throughout this country.

EXPERIMENTAL DATA IN SUPPORT OF EARLY AMBULATION

Cardiac Function. In a study of the causes of death in cardiac failure, Williams and Rainey found that the three great causes of death in patients admitted with this diagnosis were infarction of the lungs, pneumonia and uremia. Their study suggested that complete bed rest favored the development of conditions which tended to hasten death. Following these studies, Harrison found that the mortality rate was no greater for "three day cardiacs" than for "three week cardiacs," the designations referring to the time the patients were kept in bed after being admitted to the hospital in failure. Moreover, the "three day cardiacs" were happier patients. Carrying this problem to the experimental laboratory, Thomas and Harrison studied the effect of enforced immobilization on rats subjected to a standardized myocardial injury. The rats with severely restricted activity showed a higher mortality rate. They found, in general, that if one waited even so short a time as from five to seven days following cardiac injury relatively strenuous muscular exercise did not increase the mortality rate. Although Thomas and Harrison did not advocate prompt vigorous exercise following myocardial infarction in human beings, they did make a strong plea against the indiscriminate use of prolonged bed rest in patients with congestive heart failure. Since these reports, the emphasis on bed rest in the management of medical patients has gradually shifted to allow for individualization in therapy and has resulted in much more physical activity in convalescence, not only in cases of heart failure but also in many other types of disease.

Wound Healing. The large number of surgical cases mobilized immediately following operation and reported by Leithauser did much to orient surgeons to the point of view that early ambulation was not attended by more frequent or more severe complications. These clinical studies, supported by those of Powers and others, indicated that the incidence of wound disruption was not increased when early ambulation was practiced, and in the experimental laboratory Royster, McCain and Sloan showed that, following a standardized operative procedure in dogs, those animals forced to take a fixed amount of exercise daily in the postoperative period had no greater incidence of wound complications than did the controls. Their data were in substantial agreement with those reported by Newburger, and findings of this type have now been corroborated in most surgical clinics.

Pulmonary Ventilation. In 1928 Powers drew attention to the significance of the vital capacity in relation to postoperative pulmonary complications. Elevation of the diaphragm in the recumbent position, pooling of excessive tracheobronchial secretions, the disinclination of the patient to cough because of pain, and the diminished respiratory excursions following both abdominal and thoracic operations all contribute to the incidence of postoperative atelectasis and pneumonitis. Many of these processes are reversed by active exercise, and the upright position is surely more conducive to good pulmonary ventilation than is the slumped semi-Fowler position. The impression that prompt ambulation decreases the frequency of pulmonary complications is generally held throughout the country.

Phlebothrombosis and Pulmonary Embolism. Opinion differs on whether or not early ambulation decreases the incidence of venous emboli. At the Hospital of the University of Pennsylvania early activity for postoperative patients has not decreased the incidence of phlebothrombosis and pulmonary embolism (Ravdin and Kirby). The question is not easily settled, however, owing to the fact that the diagnosis in nonfatal cases can rarely be established conclusively. It has been pointed out that individuals and clinics with an active interest in this condition are apt to make the diagnosis more often and upon the basis of more minimal signs. DeBakey has recently summarized current thought on this subject and concludes simply that the problem has yet to be solved. Nevertheless, while early ambulation has not been shown to decrease venous disease, neither has it been shown to increase this condition. It may yet be shown that a most important contributing factor in the etiology of this condition is the shortened clotting and bleeding time which is a part of the alarm response.

Gastro-Intestinal Function. Postoperative distention and gas pains are less troublesome in ambulatory patients. Bowel movements are facilitated, and the abnormal strain attendant upon enemas and the unaccustomed use of a bedpan is avoided. These patients also eat more readily.

THE METABOLIC EFFECTS OF PROLONGED IMMOBILIZATION

In the foregoing paragraphs the clinical aspects of early ambulation have been touched upon. We have come to realize that these superficial manifestations represent the sum total of countless integrated cellular processes. Even yet the definition of these cellular processes lies, for the most part, beyond the bounds of present knowledge. Yet, beginnings have been made in mapping out the directions along which further and more fundamental research may reasonably be expected to proceed. Several of these investigations may be cited.

Nitrogen Balance in Normal Subjects at Bed Rest. The metabolic effects of prolonged immobilization of normal subjects in plaster casts have been studied by Deitrick, Whedon and Shorr, and moderate negative nitrogen balances were observed. There was little change in the amounts excreted during the first four days of immobilization but then there was an abrupt increase in nitrogen elimination. During the recovery stage, the nitrogen excretion remained high for a few days but then it rapidly fell to control levels and below, as nitrogen was stored. In a second study, two of the previous subjects were immobilized in casts but were placed on an oscillating rather than a fixed bed. The nitrogen losses were less than in the first study. Moreover, stiffness of the joints and muscular pains were diminished. Cuthbertson, in his observations on the nitrogen balance following fractures, found that the loss of nitrogen, calcium and phosphorus could be decreased by massage and passive motion of the injured limb.

Calcium Metabolism. In support of the clinical observation that immobilized patients are more prone to develop nephrolithiasis, Deitrick and his coworkers found that patients in casts showed on the third day of bed rest a negative calcium balance which reached a peak during the fourth to fifth week and decreased slowly in the recovery period, reaching control levels in about three weeks, and then actually storing calcium for an additional period of time. There was a corresponding negative phosphorus balance. Armstrong has emphasized that not only the fractured bone but also the normal bones are affected in the decalcification which follows a fracture or immobilization in a cast. He has

TABLE 9

Undesirable Effects of Prolonged Bed Rest

1. Muscular strength and size are diminished.
2. Postural cardiovascular reflexes are impaired.
3. The appetite is decreased.
4. Psychiatric problems increase.
5. Bowel function is sluggish.
6. Pulmonary ventilation is reduced, especially in elderly patients.
7. There is an increased incidence of renal stones.
8. There are metabolic alterations which include negative nitrogen and calcium balances.

stressed the necessity for considering the skeleton as a physiologic unit, and this concept has received abundant amplification through the use of radioisotopes in the study of bone metabolism.

The etiology of this negative calcium and phosphorus balance is not settled. A change in the level of activity of the parathyroids or in the biologic effectiveness of their secretion is of course a possibility. Also, certain individuals with thyrotoxicosis present a negative calcium balance and an osteoporosis, and thus a possible alteration in effective thyroid activity may be considered in immobilized patients. However, Deitrick and his coworkers found an average decrease of 6.9 per cent in the basal metabolic rate in their subjects at bed rest. We have also seen that osteoporosis may occur in Cushing's syndrome, but the urinary excretion of 17-ketosteroids and total corticoids was not significantly altered in the patients studied by Deitrick and his coworkers.

MUSCULAR STRENGTH AND CIRCUMFERENCE OF THE EXTREMITIES

It is common knowledge that exercise of a part results in muscle hypertrophy and, conversely, that disuse results in tissue atrophy. This is particularly striking where the leg is immobilized in a cast without exercise, but it is also observed in muscle masses following prolonged bed rest. This can be readily demonstrated by measuring the circumference of the extremity and following changes therein. This diminution in the circumference of the limb is accompanied by a decrease in muscular strength and exercise tolerance.

The basic physiologic processes whose vigor suffers following prolonged bed rest but is strengthened by physical conditioning must be revealed by newer horizons of concept and technic. Meanwhile, the clinical value of quadriceps and other exercises for extremities in casts and of early physical activity for the whole patient is established.

POSTURAL HEMODYNAMICS

Every physician is familiar with the faintness and vertigo which the patient experiences when first arising following an illness. Starr and Mayock made a very careful study of this "incoordination of the circulation" in the course of a search for objective measures which might be used to quantitate rates of convalescence. They found that on standing during the early postoperative period the pulse rate, respiration and oxygen consumption, though not unduly increased by exercise, returned to normal more slowly after operation than was the case preoperatively. Thus, the average dyspnea ratio, a measure of the prolongation of increased respiration, was increased during convalescence. Reaching a maximum in the seventh to the eleventh day after operation, the difference was statistically significant at that time; later the abnormality diminished as the patient improved. These workers concluded that whatever the exact physiologic abnormality which prevents proper adaptation to the standing position after operation may be, it is improved by practice. It took only a day or two of being up and about for the response on arising to return to normal in most cases. On the tenth day after operation those patients who were exercised and permitted out of bed from the second day onward were more normal in this respect than those who had remained in bed until the tenth day.

Most students of this problem agree that the symptoms experienced on first arising after prolonged bed rest are probably due in large measure to cerebral ischemia, and many have considered this ischemia to be the result of a poor venous return to the heart, secondary to a reduced plasma volume and to decreased muscle mass and tone. However, in many of their patients Starr and Mayock found no significant diminution in cardiac output as measured by the ballistocardiographic method.

A rewarding approach to this problem of circulatory adaptation to the upright position following operation would seem to be a study of the effect of spontaneous or induced metabolic derangements on circulatory reflexes. Starr and Mayock found the cardiac output increased in those patients whose dietary intake was increased by operation, such as in esophageal or pharyngeal carcinoma, in contrast to the findings in other patients.

THE DESIRE TO GET WELL

The concepts of all physicians have been influenced by the revelations of the past decade concerning the profound influence which the mind exerts over most physiologic processes. We now find it unrealistic to separate the "organic" from the "inorganic" in a great many of the most common diseases to which man is heir, such as "functional" gastrointestinal disease, peptic ulcer and hypertension. For this reason, it must be a planned objective to enlist the enthusiastic participation of the patient in his own convalescence.

The psychologic reorientation of both the physician toward the patient and the patient toward himself has been a major accomplishment of early ambulation. When the patient is helped out of bed the day following what he thought was an operation which would inactivate him for a considerable period of time, he quickly begins to take a certain pride in his recuperative powers, and this pride flowers under the skillful guidance of the thoughtful physician. Under such care the patient becomes increasingly extroverted, rather than introverted, and many practical and tangible advantages are derived from such a program. Limited exercise and environmental interests enhance the appetite and therewith strengthen the many processes dependent upon effective nutrition. The patient who can be helped to the bathroom is less likely to be preoccupied with dysuria or bowel dysfunctionn, and certainly the ambulatory patient is less bothered by gas pains.

The patient on prolonged bed rest frequently develops definite psychologic problems. The normal subjects studied by Deitrick, Whedon and Shorr presented definite emotional problems after variable lengths of time. These problems were manifested chiefly in the daily exchanges between these patients with the doctors and nurses, trivial real or imagined grievances being magnified beyond all proportion. These emotional disturbances were generally found to be simply exaggerations of the basic personality types represented by these subjects under normal conditions. Such side effects of enforced bed rest are well appreciated by every house officer who has cared for chronically ill patients.

The "will to live" is a quality weighed through the centuries by experienced physicians in balancing the scales of prognosis. Knowing as we now do that there exist direct pathways between the cerebral cortex and the endocrine organs which enable the organisms successfully to withstand trauma, it would seem appropriate to preserve an open mind concerning the influence which the patient's emotional status may have upon the quality of his convalescence.

REFERENCES

Allison, N., and Brooks, B.: Bone atrophy: a clinical study of the changes in bone which result from disuse. Arch. Surg., 5:499, 1922.

Armstrong, W. D.: Bone metabolism. Federation Proc., 3:201, 1944.

———: Mechanism of skeletal disuse atrophy. *Ibid.*, 5:120, 1946.

Boldt, H. J.: The management of laparotomy patients and their modified after treatment. New York Med. J., 85:145, 1907.
Castleman, B.: Pulmonary infarction and atelectasis: report of case presenting evidence of causal relationship. Arch. Path., 35:299, 1943.
Claremont, H. E.: Shortening of postoperative convalescence. Lancet, 1:427, 1922.
Coryllos, P. N., and Birnbaum, G. L.: Circulation in compressed, atelectatic and pneumonic lung. Arch. Surg., 19:1346, 1929.
Cosgriff, S. W., Diefenbach, A. F., and Vogt, W., Jr.: Hypercoagulability of the blood associated with ACTH and cortisone therapy. Am. J. Med. 9:752, 1950.
Cuthbertson, D. P.: The influence of prolonged muscular rest on the metabolism. Biochem. J., 23:1328, 1929.
DeBakey, M. E.: The problem of thrombo-embolism. Ann. Surg., 132:158, 1950.
Deitrick, J. E., Whedon, G. D., and Shorr, E.: Effects of immobilization. Am. J. Med., 4:3, 1948.
Dock, W.: The evil sequelae of bed rest. J.A.M.A., 125:1083, 1944.
Eastman, M. J.: The abuse of rest in obstetrics. J.A.M.A., 125:1077, 1944.
Ghormley, R. K.: The abuse of rest in bed in orthopedic surgery. J.A.M.A., 125:1085, 1944.
Harrison, T. R.: Abuse of rest as a therapeutic measure for patients with cardiovascular disease. J.A.M.A., 125:1075, 1944.
Howard, J. E.: Nephrolithiasis in fracture patients. Ann. Int. Med., 16:176, 1942.
Keeton, R. W., Cole, W. H., Calloway, N., Glickman, N., Mitchell, H. H., Dyniewicz, J., and Howes, D.: Convalescence: a study in the physiological recovery of nitrogen metabolism and liver function. Ann. Int. Med., 28:521, 1948.
Leithauser, D. J., and Bergo, H. L.: Early rising and ambulatory activity after operation. Arch. Surg., 42:1086, 1941.
Menninger, K.: The abuse of rest in psychiatry. J.A.M.A., 125:1087, 1944.
Nelson, E. W., and Collins, C. G.: Cotton suture material and early ambulation. Surg., Gynec. & Obst., 12:109, 1942.
Newburger, B.: Early postoperative walking: the influence of exercise on wound healing in rats. Surgery, 13:692, 1943.
———: Early postoperative walking. Ibid., 14:142, 1943.
Powers, J. H.: The abuse of rest as a therapeutic measure in surgery, J.A.M.A., 125:1079, 1944.
———: Vital capacity: its significance in relation to postoperative pulmonary complications. Arch. Surg., 17:304, 1928.
Ravdin, I. S., and Kirby, C. K.: Experiences with ligation and heparin in thromboembolic disease. Surgery, 29:334, 1951.
Ries, E.: Some radical changes in the after-treatment of celiotomy cases. J.A.M.A., 33:454, 1899.
Robertson, G.: Short hospital convalescence following common abdominal operations. Practitioner, 119:162, 1927.
Royster, H. P., McCain, L. I., and Sloan, A.: Wound healing in early ambulation. Surg., Gynec. & Obst., 86:565, 1948.
Starr, I., and Mayock, R. L.: Convalescence from surgical procedures. I. Studies of the circulation, lying and standing, of tremor, and of a program of bed exercises and early rising. Am. J. M. Sc., 210:701, 1945.
——— and Mayock, R. L.: Canvalescence from surgical procedures. II. Studies of various physiological responses to a mild exercise test. Ibid., 713.
Thomas, W. C., and Harrison, T. R.: Effect of artificial restriction of activity on recovery of rats from experimental myocardial injury. Am. J. M. Sc., 208:436, 1944.
Williams, R. H., and Rainey, J.: Cause of death in patients with congestive heart failure. Am. Heart J., 15:385, 1938.

CHAPTER 5

THE ENDOCRINOLOGY OF SURGICAL INFECTIONS, THERMAL BURNS, TISSUE REPAIR AND NEOPLASIA

SURGICAL INFECTIONS

The role of the endocrines in the management of surgical infections had scarcely been noted before the widespread use of ACTH and cortisone. To be sure, patients with panhypopituitarism, hypothyroidism or Addison's disease had long been known to be either more susceptible to, or less able to cope with, infections than are normal subjects. However, the observation by White and Dougherty that a single injection of ACTH significantly increased the serum antibody titer in previously immunized rabbits stimulated interest in this field, and recently Kass and his coworkers have reported their results with the use of ACTH and cortisone in pneumonia. They found that fever and toxic symptoms were abolished even where the blood culture remained positive for pneumococci. Thus, there was no evidence of a bactericidal effect, and the date of the appearance and the magnitude of the rise in antipneumococcal antibodies and cold agglutinins were unaffected by the ACTH and cortisone. There was also no evidence of an effect on the rate of resolution of consolidated lobes. These authors suggested that the beneficial effect of ACTH resulted from the effect of the adrenal steroids on the metabolic processes which are active in the cellular response to infection.

There are other inflammatory processes, particularly those with an allergic component, which are benefited by ACTH or cortisone therapy. We have recently observed a case of extremely severe exfoliative dermatitis caused by pencillin which responded almost miraculously to ACTH therapy when all other treatment had proved inefficacious.

It is too early properly to assess the future of steroid therapy in surgical infections, but experiences such as these indicate new points of departure for the investigation of immunologic relationships between the bacterium and the host.

THERMAL BURNS

The effects of ACTH and cortisone on tissue reaction and infections following thermal injury have been the subject of a number of provocative reports. Whitelaw and Mulholland were impressed with the apparent efficacy of these agents in decreasing infection, pain and fluid loss and in enabling homologous skin grafts to take and survive. However, other workers have not been able to demonstrate the survival of skin grafts taken from another person, and Evans has not observed that the general course of the burn patient is materially improved by such therapy. All agree that further study is necessary.

THE EFFECTS OF HORMONES ON TISSUE REPAIR AND REGENERATION

Anterior Pituitary Growth Hormone. In 1941 Cuthbertson, Shaw and Young studied the effect of an extract of the anterior lobe of the pituitary gland on the rate of wound healing, but no significant effect was demonstrated. Yet, in the light of the more recent demonstration by Friedberg and Greenberg that both normal and hypophysectomized rats exhibit a greater uptake by muscle protein of methionine labeled with radioactive sulfur following injection of these animals with the growth hormone, it may be advisable to re-open this question for further investigation with isotopic methods.

The Thyroid. In 1945 Diaz-Guerrero and his associates found that delayed denervation atrophy and neuromuscular regeneration were obtained in thiouracil-treated rats following nerve crush injury. The injection of thyroxine accelerated both atrophy and regeneration, and it is not unlikely that these altered rates of cellular activity were related to the decreased mitotic activity found by Fleischmann and Breckler in the corneas of hypothyroid rats. Drabkin has demonstrated a significant influence of the thyroid secretion on the cytochrome C content of all tissues, an effect which suggests a mechanism whereby thyroxine helps to regulate the oxygen consumption of the various organs. Thyroidectomy or the administration of thiouracil decreased the cytochrome C content of the tissues. Under these conditions the rate of liver regeneration was less than normal but was not greatly retarded.

The Adrenal Cortex. There have been conflicting reports concerning the effect of ACTH and cortisone on wound healing. Howes and his associates investigated this problem in animals and gained the definite impression that the administration of these agents in large doses did retard wound healing. Cole and his coworkers, in a histologic study of wound healing and its relationship to cortisone and serum antihyaluronidase, concluded that the effects of cortisone on healing wounds were not striking and that the in vivo inhibition of hyaluronidase by cortisone observed by other workers was not due to an alteration in the normal serum antihyaluronidase by cortisone. Thomas and Rhoads have examined the effect of cortisone on wound healing in rabbits, but they have not demonstrated a consistent deleterious effect on fibroblastic proliferation. However, Ingle and his associates found that ACTH inhibited somatic growth in male rats. This finding has to be reconciled with the report of Berman and his coworkers that the adrenal steroids aid hepatic regeneration. These investigators showed that adrenalectomy resulted in a marked depression of liver regeneration following partial hepatectomy.

Clearly, the effects of abnormal concentrations of the adrenocortical steroids on wound healing remain to be defined. Meanwhile, it may be remembered that "physiologic" increases in the amounts of these substances, elaborated following injury, have in the past been compatible with satisfactory wound healing.

THE ENDOCRINOLOGY OF NEOPLASIA

A number of neoplastic diseases are now known to be markedly affected by alterations in hormonal relationships, and the effects of specific hormones on certain malignant processes have quickened interest in the medical treatment of cancer.

The Pituitary. None of the pituitary hormones has so far been shown to be important in the etiology of cancer. The absence of pituitary hormones seems to retard but not to arrest malignant growth (Selye). The effects of ACTH on lymphoid tumors will be discussed in connection with the influence of the adrenal cortex on neoplasia.

The Thyroid. The thyroid may indirectly influence neoplastic processes by virtue of its regulation of rates of metabolism, growth, differentiation of tissues, distribution of colloids, neuromuscular activity, circulatory performance, tolerance to certain drugs, gastro-intestinal function, and the formation of blood. However, thyroxine appears to have no direct carcinogenic or anticarcinogenic action.

The Adrenal Cortex. White and Dougherty showed that an increased adrenocortical secretion resulted in the rapid dissolution of lymph nodes, and Heilman and Kendall noted that the administration of compound E was followed by a regression of lymphoid tumors in mice. With these observations in mind, Pearson and his associates administered ACTH and cortisone to patients with lymphoid tumors and found a rapid regression in the size of the lymph nodes. Unfortunately, this regression was not a permanent one, but these studies have been most useful in suggesting new approaches to the study of malignancy.

Dobriner and his associates have reported a series of prolonged and exacting studies on the urinary excretion of ketosteroid fractions in cancer patients. They discovered in such individuals an abnormal alpha-ketosteroid fraction. This compound was found in lymphocytic leukemia and in carcinomas of the breast, prostate and larynx. Although it was found in one apparently normal person, this subject later developed carcinoma of the breast. These workers believe that their results most likely indicate an abnormality of the adrenocortical secretion in certain patients harboring malignancy, and it may be hoped that once the exact nature of the deranged function is established it will be possible to correct it.

Estrogens. These streoids were among the earliest hormonal agents implicated in the etiology of cancer. In 1938 Gardner, Allen, Smith and Strong noted the development of cervical carcinoma in mice receiving estrogens. The following year Laccasagne reported that the administration of estradiol was associated with the development of mammary carcinoma in male mice of a susceptible strain. He concluded that either the estrogen was directly the cause of the malignant growth or it indirectly effected this end result by causing the hypertrophy of an organ in which other factors later produced carcinoma. That same year Allaben and Owen reported a case of adenocarcinoma of the breast which had followed a year of continuous estrogen therapy. Since then many investigators have been able to produce malignant neoplasms of the breast in male mice of susceptible strains by the use of estrogen therapy. It has also been possible to lower the age level at which susceptible strains develop malignancy. Nevertheless, the precise relationship between estrogens and mammary and uterine carcinoma in human beings has not been settled.

The regression of uterine fibroids following the menopause had long been appreciated clinically when, in 1941, Lipschutz and Vargas induced uterine and extragenital fibroids in guinea pigs by the prolonged administration of estrogens.

Estrogens have also been implicated in the genesis of certain tumors of the testis. In 1940 Bonser and Robson, and Hooker, Gardner and Pfeiffer reported the production of metastasizing testicular tumors in the Strong A strain of mice. There was evidence that some of these tumors secreted an androgenic material.

The palliative effects of estrogenic or androgenic therapy in mammary and other types of cancer are more fully discussed in the chapter on endocrine therapy, but it may be mentioned here that these effects are often quite gratifying.

Testosterone. Since Huggins and his associates reported the remarkable regression exhibited by advanced prostatic carcinoma with metastases following castration in such patients, the beneficial effects of this operation and/or estrogen therapy have been established. In view of the fact that the prostate does not develop normally in castrates or eunuchs, it is clear that testosterone is of importance in supporting the normal growth of this organ. Moore believes that both benign hypertrophy and carcinoma of the prostate are caused by an imbalance of the endocrinologic status of the patient. The administration of estrogenic substances, even in the absence of castration, influences the hormonal balance favorably and often is followed by a regression of advanced prostatic carcinoma.

Gardner, Dougherty and Williams have reported that testosterone propionate inhibits the tendency of mice receiving estradiol to develop lymphosarcoma.

Progesterone. Hertz has recently reported striking regression of advanced carcinomas of the cervix following progesterone therapy.

To summarize, there has been a great increase in interest concerning the effects of various hormones on neoplastic growth. Broadly speaking, these influences are effected through an alteration of previously existing hormonal balances. These altered endocrine relationships in turn promote a metabolic response which is unfavorable for the growth of neoplastic cells. These effects upon the metabolism of the host are likely mediated through the hormonal regulation of enzymatic activity. The enzymes concerned will be the subject of intensive investigation in the years to come.

REFERENCES

Allaben, G. R., and Owen, G. E.: Adenocarcinoma of the breast coincidental with strenuous endocrine therapy. J.A.M.A., *112*:1933, 1939.

Ball, H. A., and Samuels, L. T.: The relation of the hypophysis to the growth of malignant tumors. Am. J. Cancer, 26:547, 1936.

Berman, D., Sylvester, M., Hay, E. C., and Selye, H.: The adrenal and early hepatic regeneration. Endocrinology, *41*:258, 1947.

Bonser, G. M., and Robson, J. M.: The effects of prolonged estrogen administration upon male mice of various strains: development of testicular tumors in the Strong A strain. J. Path. & Bact., *51*:9, 1940.

Chase, J. H., White, A., and Dougherty, T. F.: Enhancement of circulating antibody concentration by adrenal cortical hormones. J. Immunol., 52:101, 1946.

Cole, J., Orbison, J. L., Holden, W. B., Hancock, T., Lindsay, J. L., Ankeney, J. L., and Hubay, C. A.: A histological study of wound healing and its relationship to cortisone and serum antihyaluronidase; in American College of Surgeons: Surgical Forum (Proceedings of the Forum Sessions, Thirty-Sixth Clinical Congress of the American College of Surgeons). Philadelphia, W. B. Saunders Company, 1951, p. 443.

Colebrook, L.: A New Approach to the Treatment of Burns and Scalds. London, Fine Technical Publications, 1950.

Cook, E. S., and Fardon, J. C.: Wound hormone concept. Surg., Gynec. & Obst., 75: 220, 1942.

Cuthbertson, D. P., Shaw, G. B., and Young, F. G.: Anterior pituitary gland and protein metabolism; influence of anterior pituitary extract on rate of healing. J. Endocrinol., *2*:475, 1941.

Diaz-Guerrero, R., Thompson, J. D., and Hines, H. M.: Effect of thymectomy, hyperthyroidism and hypothyroidism on neuromuscular atrophy and regeneration. Am. J. Physiol., *151*:91, 1945.

Dobriner, K., Gordon, E., Rhoads, C. P., Lieberman, S., and Fieser, L. F.: Steroid hormone excretion by normal and pathological individuals. Science, 95:534, 1942

———, Rhoads, C. P., Lieberman, S., Hill, B. R., and Fieser, L. F.: Abnormal alpha ketosteroid excretion in patients with neoplastic disease. *Ibid.*, 99:494, 1944.

Dougherty, T. F., and White, A.: Effect of pituitary adrenotropic hormone on lymphoid tissue. Proc. Soc. Exper. Biol. & Med., 53:132, 1943.

———, Chase, J. H., and White, A.: Demonstration of antibodies in lymphocytes. *Ibid.*, 58:135, 1945.

Drabkin, D. L.: The effect of thyroidectomy and thiouracil on cytochrome C metabolism and liver regeneration. Federation Proc., 7:151, 1948.

Ellison, E. H., Martin, B. C., Williams, R. D., Clatworthy, H. W., Hamwi, G., and Zollinger, R. M.: The effect of ACTH and cortisone on the survival of homologous skin grafts. Ann. Surg., *134*:495, 1951.

Evans, E. I.: Personal communication.
—— and Butterfield, W. J. H.: The stress response in the severely burned. Ann. Surg., *134*:588, 1951.
Findley, C. W., and Howes, E. L.: Potassium and wound healing. Surgery, *28*:970, 1950.
Fleischmann, W., and Breckler, I. A.: Mitotic and wound healing activities of the corneal epithelium in thiouracil treated and thyroidectomized rats. Endocrinology, *41*:266, 1947.
Friedberg, F., and Greenberg, D. M.: Endocrine regulation of amino acid levels in blood and tissues. J. Biol. Chem., *168*:405, 1947.
Gardner, W. V., Allen, E., Smith, G. M., and Strong, L. C.: Carcinoma of the cervix of mice receiving estrogens. J.A.M.A., *110*:1182, 1938.
——, Dougherty, T. F., and Williams, W. L.: Lymphoid tumors in mice receiving steroid hormones. Cancer Research, *4*:73, 1944.
Harvey, S. C., and Howes, E. L.: Effect of high protein diet on the growth of fibroblasts. Ann. Surg., *91*:641, 1930.
Heilman, F. R., and Kendall, E. C.: The influence of 11-dehydro-17-hydroxycorticosterone (compound E) on the growth of a malignant tumor in the mouse. Endocrinology, *34*:416, 1944.
Heppel, L. A.: The electrolytes of muscle and liver in potassium depleted rats. Am. J. Physiol., *127*:385, 1939.
Hertz, R.: Progesterone and carcinoma of the cervix; in Laurentian Hormone Conference, 1950. (Personal communication.)
Hooker, C. W., Gardner, W. V., and Pfeiffer, C. O.: Testicular tumors in mice receiving estrogens. J.A.M.A., *115*:443, 1940.
Howes, E. L., Plotz, C. M., Blunt, J. W., and Ragan, C.: Retardation of wound healing by cortisone. Surgery, *28*:177, 1950.
Huggins, C., Stevens, R. E., and Hodges, C. V.: Studies on prostatic cancer. II. The effects of castration on advanced carcinoma of prostate gland. Arch. Surg., *43*:209, 1941.
Ingle, D. J., Prestrud, M. C., Li, C. H., and Evans, H. M.: The relationship of diet to the effect of adrenocorticotrophic hormone upon urinary nitrogen, glucose and electrolytes. Endocrinology, *41*:170, 1947.
Kass, E. H., Ingbar, S. H., and Finland, M.: Effects of adrenocorticotropic hormone in pneumonia: clinical, bacteriological and serological studies. Ann. Int. Med., *33*: 1081, 1950.
Kobak, M. W., Benditt, E. P., Wissler, R. W., and Steffie, C. H.: The relation of protein deficiency to experimental wound healing. Surg., Gynec. & Obst., *85*:751, 1947.
Kochakian, C. D.: Anabolic effects of steroid hormones. Vitamins & Hormones, *4*:255, 1946.
Kozoll, D. D., Hoffman, W. S., and Meyer, K. A.: Nitrogen balance studies on surgical patients receiving amino acids; observations on patients with obstructing lesions of the esophagus and stomach receiving amino acids by parenteral injection as the exclusive source of protein. Arch. Surg., *51*:59, 1945.
Kramer, B., and Tisdall, F. F.: The distribution of sodium, potassium, calcium, and magnesium between the corpuscles of serum and human blood. J. Biol. Chem., *53*:241, 1922.
Laccasagne, A.: Relationship of hormones and mammary adenocarcinoma in the mouse. Am. J. Cancer, *37*:414, 1939.
Lerman, J.: The endocrine activity of thyroid tumors and the influence of the thyroid hormone on tumors in general; in Endocrinology of Neoplastic Diseases. New York, Oxford University Press, 1947, p. 392.
Lieberman, S., Dobriner, K., Hill, B. R., Fieser, L. F., and Rhoads, C. P.: Studies in steroid metabolism. II. Identification and characterizations of ketosteroids isolated from urine of healthy and diseased persons. J. Biol. Chem., *172*:263, 1948.
Lipschutz, A., and Vargas, L., Jr.: Structure and origin of uterine and extragenital fibroids induced experimentally in the guinea pig by prolonged administration of estrogens. Cancer Research, *1*:236, 1941.
Localio, S. A., Chassin, J. L., and Hinton, J. W.: Tissue protein depletion; factor in wound disruption. Surg., Gynec. & Obst., *86*:107, 1948.

Lund, C. C., and Crandon, J. H.: Nutrition as it affects healing. M. Clin. North America, 27:561, 1943.
Menkin, V.: Studies on inflammation. J. Exper. Med., 64:485, 1936.
Moore, R. A.: Benign hypertrophy and carcinoma of the prostate; in Endocrinology of Neoplastic Diseases. New York, Oxford University Press, 1947, p. 208.
Mudge, G. H., and Vislocky, K.: Electrolyte changes in human striated muscle in acidosis and alkalosis. J. Clin. Investigation, 28:482, 1949.
Mulholland, J. H.: Personal communication.
Paul, H. E., Paul, M. F., Taylor, J. D., and Marsters, R.: Biochemistry of wound healing. II. Water and protein content of healing tissue of skin wounds. Arch. Biochem., 17:269, 1948.
Parsons, W. W., and McCall, E. F.: The role of estrogenic substances in the production of malignant mammary lesions, with report of case of adenocarcinoma of the breast, possibly induced by strenuous estrogen therapy. Surgery, 9:780, 1941.
Pearson, O. H., Eliel, L. P., Rawson, R. W., Dobriner, K., and Rhoads, C. P.: ACTH- and cortisone-induced regression of lymphoid tumors. Cancer, 2:943, 1949.
Ravdin, I. S.: Nitrogen balance. Surgery, 24:1035, 1948.
Reiss, M.: Lactogenic hormone and fat metabolism. J. Endocrinol., 5:xxxv, 1947.
─────: The pituitary-adrenocortical relationship. Ibid., xli.
Rhoads, C. P., Dobriner, K., Gordon, E., Fieser, L. F., and Lieberman, S.: Metabolic studies on the urinary excretion of steroids in normals, in patients with adrenal hyperplasia, and in cancer patients. Tr. A. Am. Physicians, 57:203, 1942.
Roy, A.: Influence of hormones on growth in rats. The galactopoietic activity of hormones in cows in declining lactation. J. Endocrinol., 5:xxxv, 1947.
Selye, H.: Experimental investigations concerning the role of the pituitary in tumorigenesis; in Endocrinology of Neoplastic Diseases. New York, Oxford University Press, 1947, p. 45.
Thomas, J., and Rhoads, J. E.: Personal communication.
Twombly, G. H.: Breast cancer produced in male mice of the C57 (Black) strain of Little. Proc. Soc. Exper. Biol. & Med., 44:617, 1940.
Waugh, W. G.: Systemic factors influencing healing. Brit. M. J., 2:236, 1941.
Weisman, P. A., Quinby, W. C., Wight, A., and Cannon, B.: The adrenal cortical hormones and homografting: exploration of a concept. Ann. Surg., 134:506, 1951.
White, A., and Dougherty, T. F.: The role of lymphocytes in normal and immune globulin production and the mode of release of globulin from lymphocytes. Ann. New York Acad. Sc., 46:859, 1946.
Whitelaw, M. J.: Physiologic reaction to ACTH in severe burns. J.A.M.A., 144:678, 1950.
Williams, R. H., Jaffe, H., and Kemp, C.: Effect of severe stress upon thyroid function. Am. J. Physiol., 155:291, 1949.

CHAPTER 6

ENDOCRINE THERAPY IN SURGICAL PATIENTS

Although hormonal therapy in surgical patients is still in its infancy, certain practical applications have already been established. These proved indications will be presented in some detail, and other less crystallized trends will be mentioned. Obviously, a full scale review of substitution therapy in conditions such as hypothyroidism, absolute hypoadrenalism (Addison's disease), hypoinsulinism (diabetes mellitus), and hypopituitarism is beyond the length of this volume. While these conditions are frequently encountered and treated by the surgeon, they are more properly managed by the internist, and hypoparathyroidism has been discussed under complications of thyroidectomy. Thus, the following will be considered:

A. Absolute and Relative Adrenocortical Insufficiency in Patients Undergoing Surgery
B. Drug Sensitivities and Exfoliative Dermatitis
C. Management of the Diabetic Patient Subjected to Surgery
D. Hormonal Therapy in Malignancy
E. Use of Androgens to Increase Nitrogen Retention and Muscular Strength
F. Therapeutic Uses of Posterior Pituitary Hormones

ABSOLUTE AND RELATIVE ADRENOCORTICAL INSUFFICIENCY IN PATIENTS COMING TO SURGERY

Absolute Insufficiency

Patients with severe Addison's disease who require operative intervention are not common, but when this situation presents itself it is a most exacting one with which to deal. If the surgical pathology is such as to permit an elective procedure, the problem is more easily managed. During the three days prior to operation the patient should receive 25 mg. of cortisone by mouth every six hours and 5 mg. of DOCA intramuscularly daily. Thorn and his associates advise the administration of an additional 10 mg. of DOCA (2 cc.) intramuscularly on the morning of operation. Liberal amounts of all vitamins, particularly C and K, are given for several days preoperatively and continued postoperatively. Antibiotics are begun on admission and continued through convalescence. At least one hour prior to the beginning of anesthesia an intravenous drip of 10 per cent glucose in physiologic saline solution is begun, and to it are added 50 cc. of aqueous adrenocortical extract. Throughout the operation hypotension is combatted with additional injections of ACE, plasma, and whole blood transfusions, and the careful use of epinephrine and/or neosynephrine. At the end of the operation the patient's condition is evaluated and therapy is decided upon as needed. Additional saline should be given with caution, since too much salt and water in conjunction with large amounts of DOCA may precipitate heart failure.

The anesthesia of choice is local. The ideal general anesthetic is one which is quickly effective and rapidly eliminated. Morphine and the long-acting barbiturates are poorly tolerated.

In the postoperative period the administration of 25 mg. of cortisone intramuscularly every six to twelve hours may be adequate to maintain the patient. This can be supplemented with 5 mg. of DOCA intramuscularly daily, care being exercised to avoid excessive fluid retention. The patient's course should be followed by means of his symptoms, general appearance, blood pressure, blood urea nitrogen, fasting blood sugar and serum electrolytes. In an emergency the whole adrenal extract is probably still to be preferred, since its action is rapid and large doses are well tolerated. In general, we consider it more satisfactory to maintain blood pressure with adequate amounts of adrenocortical substitution therapy than to depend too heavily on such drugs as neosynephrine. The efficacy of these sympathomimetic agents in combatting sudden and precipitous falls in blood pressure in patients with adrenocortical insufficiency may be dramatic, but the writer has been associated with one such case in which the hypertension which resulted precipitated a stroke which eventuated in death.

If the patient must be operated upon in an emergency, large doses of aqueous cortical extract will serve as the bedrock of maintenance, supplemented by DOCA, cortisone, intravenous glucose and saline, and whole blood transfusions.

The outline of management offered above may be used as a tentative guide, but each patient must be followed from hour to hour and from day to day, and therapy must be given as necessary to maintain the blood pressure and other manifestations of adrenocortical sufficiency.

Relative Adrenocortical Insufficiency

This condition is far more common than was previously supposed. Many patients have adrenocortical activity that is subnormal but which is adequate for their usual pursuits. However, when these individuals are subjected to major surgical procedures their adrenocortical activity is inadequate to meet the increased metabolic need for these hormones, and signs of adrenal failure may appear. These manifestations are most likely to intervene during the operation itself or during the first forty-eight hours thereafter, since this is the period when the body needs are greatest. The most prominent of these manifestations is a fall in blood pressure, but at times it may be most difficult to determine the etiology of the hypotension observed. Thorn and his associates suggest that, since in the normal patient the circulating eosinophils almost disappear from the blood stream within the first twelve hours following operation, a total eosinophil count as high as 50 to 100 cells per cu. mm. during the first twenty-four hours postoperatively indicates adrenocortical insufficiency. Treatment should consist of ACE and/or cortisone in adequate doses. An initial dose of 50 cc. of cortical extract intramuscularly or intravenously should be followed by 25 mg. of cortisone intramuscularly every six hours, later reduced to 12.5 mg. by mouth every six hours. It has been conclusively demonstrated in a number of centers that cortisone is effective orally, and this route of administration should be employed when possible. In very acute adrenocortical insufficiency the administration of DOCA would be of less importance, since time would not have permitted either marked fluid and salt loss or shifts between the intracellular and extracellular compartments.

A most important group of patients in whom to suspect latent adrenocortical insufficiency are those with active tuberculosis. Tuberculosis of the adrenals is the greatest single cause of adrenocortical insufficiency, and the current striking increase in pulmonary resections for cavitary and other types of pulmonary tuberculosis has spotlighted our present inability to predict which of these patients are best able to withstand the operation. In such patients the adrenocortical reserve can be estimated by means of a preoperative ACTH-eosinophil test as described by Thorn and his associates. In brief, a fasting total eosinophil count is performed on venous blood and 25 mg. of ACTH is then administered intramuscularly, followed by another count at the end of four hours. If the total count is diminished by as much as 50 per cent, the patient very likely has a normal adrenocortical reserve. If the total eosinophil count does not decrease by 50 per cent, however, borderline adrenocortical reserve must be suspected and the patient must be managed accordingly. Supplementary cortisone, ACE and DOCA may be administered before, during and following operation.

At times the adrenocortical insufficiency may be of pituitary origin. That is, the integrity of the adrenal cortex may be relatively unimpaired but the ACTH stimulus from the anterior lobe of the pituitary is inadequate. This condition can be diagnosed qualitatively by means of the epinephrine-eosinophil test. The technic is much the same as with the ACTH test, with the exception that the stimulus is 0.3 mg. of epinephrine. This effects the release of ACTH by the anterior pituitary. If the fall in the total eosinophil count at the end of four hours is less than 50 per cent of the control level, pituitary dysfunction is to be suspected.

Under these circumstances either ACTH or cortisone could be used as treatment for the adrenal insufficiency. In primary adrenal failure, however, ACTH would of course be of little benefit.

MANAGEMENT OF DRUG SENSITIVITIES, INCLUDING EXFOLIATIVE DERMATITIS

In few other fields have the effects of ACTH and cortisone been more striking than in that of allergy. Asthmatic patients are often greatly improved and nasal polyps may be seen to regress rapidly over a period of two or three days (Harvey). In the province of the surgeon, drug rashes frequently disappear in a matter of twenty-four to forty-eight hours. A case of exfoliative dermatitis with which we were associated responded dramatically to ACTH therapy where all other measures had failed and death seemed almost certain. Similar results have been obtained by others. The dosage which we have employed is 25 mg. of cortisone or of ACTH every six hours for the first two or three days, then 12.5 mg. every twelve hours for as long as seemed advisable. At times as much as 200 to 300 mg. has been given during the first two days of therapy. The cortisone is administered orally where possible.

MANAGEMENT OF THE DIABETIC PATIENT SUBJECTED TO SURGERY

The patient with controlled diabetes now withstands surgery so successfully that it is difficult to convince medical students that a sudden shortage of insulin and/or antibiotics could abruptly alter this happy circumstance. This achievement has been the result of intimate teamwork between the surgeon and the internist. Certain internists with special interest and background in the management of diabetes have long taken the view that diabetes mellitus is an additional indication for, rather than a contraindication to, surgical intervention. Accordingly, we have not hesitated to operate when necessary.

When possible the diabetes should be completely controlled before proceeding with the operation. To permit this a gangrenous extremity may be packed in ice for twenty-four or even forty-eight hours. Suppurative lesions elsewhere may not lend themselves to such management, and under such circumstances the diabetes is more easily controlled if the pus is drained promptly.

We prefer to operate upon these patients in the morning. Breakfast is omitted, but the patient is given one-half his usual dose of protamine insulin, if he has been on such a regimen. A slow infusion of 5 per cent glucose in 0.85 per cent saline containing 10 to 20 units of crystalline insulin is then begun. This solution is infused throughout the operation and for the remainder of the day. Approximately 2 to 3 liters is administered, but less saline may be used where this is considered advisable. The patient is returned to his normal diet and insulin the following day, or as soon as possible thereafter. Throughout the postoperative period the blood and urine sugar levels and the carbon dioxide combining power of the serum are followed closely. As long as the acid-base balance is satisfactory and the glucose levels only moderately elevated, the patient is considered to be adequately treated. No attempt should be made to keep the blood sugar normal or the urine sugar-free, for this will frequently result in hypoglycemic shocks. Under the conditions of anesthesia and operation, fairly wide and often unpredictable variations in the blood sugar levels may be expected. If the operation cannot be performed in the morning, the patient is given a liquid breakfast and the intravenous glucose, saline and insulin are begun later. The amount of insulin added to each liter of fluid is governed by the severity of the diabetes.

Diabetic Coma. The management of this condition is beyond the scope of this discussion, but it must be treated before extensive surgery is attempted. We simply suggest that in the management of the more severe diabetic states it is more often too little, rather than too much, insulin that is given. Several hundred units may be required in the first three to six hours of therapy. In addition, liberal amounts of sodium chloride and vitamins should be administered. While the initial serum potassium level may be high, as the patient is hydrated and the insulin promotes glycogen (and potassium) deposition in the liver the serum potassium may fall to dangerously low levels. Such changes may be followed by actual measurement of serum potassium levels or by observing the alterations in serial electrocardiograms. The first method is vastly superior to the second.

HORMONAL THERAPY IN ADVANCED MALIGNANCY
Carcinoma of the Prostate

Castration. The work of Huggins and his associates has established the efficacy of this operation as a palliative therapy for advanced prostatic cancer with metastases. In their now classic study of twenty-one cases in which castration was performed, four died within eight months of operation, in two the operation was too recent to permit evaluation, and in fifteen cases prompt clinical improvement occurred. Improvement was evidenced by a decrease in serum acid phosphatase in all but two cases, an increase in weight and a return of appetite, an increase in the red cells of the peripheral blood, a decrease in the amount of pain from the primary or the metastatic lesions, a shrinkage in the primary lesion, an increased density of metastatic lesions visualized by roentgenogram and, in one case, an improvement in neurologic signs of compression of the cauda equina by metastases. Untoward symptoms were a moderate swelling of the ankles, prompt abolition of sexual capacity and the development of hot flashes, the last being relieved by the administration of estrogens. A recrudescence of pain could be effected by the administration of androgens (e.g., testosterone).

This reversal of the downward course of patients with advanced prostatic cancer is, unfortunately, only temporary. While the remission in a given patient may last from a few months to several years, the average duration being about fifteen months, eventually the disease escapes from the suppressive effect of the metabolic alterations induced by castration (and/or estrogen therapy) and this turn of events is frequently heralded by a return of pain and a rise in the serum acid phosphatase level.

Estrogen Therapy. In addition to castration, or in lieu of this procedure if the patient refuses operation, palliation of advanced prostatic carcinoma may also be secured through the administration of estrogens. Whereas the relief following castration is prompt, that obtained with diethylstilbestrol is more gradual. A dosage of 5 mg. three times a day may be employed, but care must be exercised to avoid excessive fluid retention lest heart failure be precipitated.

The mechanisms whereby castration and stilbestrol effect their improvement in advanced prostatic malignancy are unknown. As a practical point in prognosis, it is worth remembering that the serum acid phosphatase level varies with the course of the disease, falling as the beneficial effects of castration and estrogen therapy are realized and rising again as the efficacy of this therapy begins to wane.

Advanced Mammary Carcinoma

Testosterone Therapy. In 1896 Beatson first suggested castration as a treatment of advanced mammary carcinoma in premenopausal women. Since that time endocrine therapy for this disease has received much attention and has proved to be of definite benefit in some patients. The studies of Adair and his associates and of Nathanson in this field have been outstanding.

As with endocrine therapy for prostatic cancer, these hormonal substances are only palliative in breast cancer. In premenopausal women androgens only are administered, since estrogens may actually enhance the growth of the tumor. For this reason it is frequently advisable to castrate the patient surgically or with irradiation (we prefer the former because of its certainty), and this castration may serve to give symptomatic relief for a period of time. If this is of no benefit or if symptoms recur, testosterone propionate may be administered in doses of 100 mg. intramuscularly three times a week. Adair found that an average cumulative dose of 3000 mg. was required before objective improvement in skeletal metastases was noted. He found that such therapy produced objective improvement in 19 per cent of forty-eight patients with skeletal metastases and in 15 per cent of fifty-four patients with extraskeletal metastases. Temporary relief of pain was obtained in forty-four of fifty-eight patients in whom this was the initial complaint. It was particularly significant that certain patients were symptomatically improved even in the presence of progression of the disease.

In the administration of androgens care must be taken to avoid dangerous elevations in the serum calcium level. The serum calcium level may be somewhat elevated even at the time testosterone therapy is begun, but if the level begins to rise under therapy the hormone should be stopped at once. Treatment may be repeated if symptoms reappear. Also, excessive fluid retention caused by this therapy may cause cardiac decompensation.

Estrogen Therapy. The criteria for the administration of estrogens in advanced breast cancer are somewhat different from the indications for androgen therapy (testosterone). Whereas androgens have their greatest effect on osseous metastases in premenopausal women, estrogens have their major beneficial effect on soft tissue lesions in postmenopausal women. Lesions of the skin, lymph nodes, pleurae and breasts may be expected to show improvement in roughly one-fourth of the patients with this type of disease. The dosage of diethylstilbestrol employed varies from 5 to 20 mg. per day, with the average dose being about 15 mg. (by mouth). Adair and his associates found it necessary to administer approximately 630 mg. before the average patient obtained relief, which lasted from two to seventeen months. Pain was relieved in slightly more than half the patients with this complaint.

Like testosterone, stilbestrol and other estrogens increase fluid retention and must be used with caution in persons with heart disease. Patients so treated frequently experience a definite improvement in their general physical condition. Their sense of well-being is enhanced, blood formation is increased, appetite is improved, and most patients gain weight. Unfortunately, early recurrence of symptoms is the rule.

Carcinoma of the Uterine Cervix

In a recent study, Hertz has obtained evidence that the administration of 250 mg. of progesterone daily for six weeks may result in a regression in advanced cancer of the uterine cervix, and that the operability rate in these patients may be increased.

Lymphoid Tumors

In 1949 Pearson and his associates reported their experience with the treatment of certain lymphoid tumors with ACTH and cortisone. Frequently the enlarged nodes literally melted over the course of two or three days, and markedly elevated white counts fell to within normal limits. Similar findings have been observed by the hematologists at the Hospital of the University of Pennsylvania. Lymphocytic leukemia is almost specifically affected by such therapy, myelogenous leukemia usually being refractory. However, such remissions are temporary and early recurrence is the rule.

General Implications

From the foregoing discussion it will again be noted that the net effect of endocrine therapy is to alter the pre-existing hormonal balance. In prostatic cancer the effect of therapy is to reduce the androgens (upon which normal prostatic growth depends) and to increase the estrogens. In mammary carcinoma the treatment varies according to whether the patient is premenopausal or postmenopausal. In postmenopausal women recurrence of symptoms following previously effective treatment with estrogens may occasionally be relieved by the administration of androgens.

USE OF TESTOSTERONE TO INCREASE NITROGEN RETENTION

There is now abundant evidence that testosterone will promote a positive nitrogen balance. Albright suggested such therapy in 1942 and Sprague, Mason and Power have recently found that the negative nitrogen balance caused by the administration of 200 mg. of cortisone per day is completely reversed by the injection of 25 mg. of testosterone propionate daily. Other workers have noted similar effects of this hormone. A suggested dosage regimen for increasing the nitrogen retention and general sense of well-being of chronically debilitated patients and paraplegics is the injection of 25 mg. of testosterone propionate two to three times weekly, or the oral use of 30 mg. of methyltestosterone daily.

POSTERIOR PITUITARY EXTRACTS

Pitocin has been widely used to stimulate uterine contraction and thus minimize postpartum hemorrhage.

Pitressin injected intramuscularly is of some value in relieving postoperative intestinal distention. It is also useful in the management of diabetes insipidus.

REFERENCES

Adair, F. E., and Herrmann, J. B.: The use of testosterone propionate in the treatment of advanced carcinoma of the breast. Ann. Surg., *123*:1023, 1946.

———, Mellors, R. C., Farrow, J. H., Woodard, H. Q., Escher, G. C., and Urban, J. A.: The use of estrogens and androgens in advanced mammary cancer. J.A.M.A., *140*: 1193, 1949.

Albright, F.: [Discussions]; in Transactions of the Conference on Bone and Wound Healing (Metabolic Aspects of Convalescence), Second Meeting, New York, December 11, 1942. New York, Josiah Macy, Jr. Foundation [n.d.], *passim*.

Auchincloss, H., and Haagensen, C. D.: Cancer of the breast possibly induced by estrogenic substance. J.A.M.A., *114*:1517, 1940.

Beatson, G. T.: On the treatment of inoperable cases of carcinoma of the mamma; suggestions for a new method of treatment with illustrative cases. Lancet, *104*:162, 1896.

Dean, A. L., Woodard, H. Q., and Twombly, G. H.: The endocrine treatment of carcinoma of the prostate. J. Urol., *49*:108, 1943.

Harvey, A. M.: The effect of ACTH and cortisone on certain allergic diseases (Mary Scott Newbold Lecture). Tr. & Stud. Coll. Physicians, Philadelphia, *19*: No. 2, 39, 1951.

Hertz, R.: Laurentian Hormone Conference, 1950. (Personal communication.)
Huggins, C.: Endocrine substances in the treatment of cancer. J.A.M.A., *141:*750, 1949.
———, Stevens, R. E., and Hodges, C. V.: Studies on prostatic cancer. II. The effects of castration on advanced carcinoma of the prostate gland. Arch. Surg., *43:*209, 1941.
Karnofsky, D. A., and Burchenal, J. H.: Present status of clinical cancer chemotherapy. Am. J. Med., *8:*767, 1950.
Nathanson, I. T.: The relationship of hormones to diseases of the breast; in Endocrinology of Neoplastic Diseases. New York, Oxford University Press, 1947, p. 171.
———, Adair, F. E., Allen, W. M., and Engle, E. T.: Estrogens and androgens in mammary cancer. J.A.M.A., *35:*987, 1947.
———, Adair, F. E., Allen, W. M., Engle, E. T., and Huggins, C.: Current status of hormone therapy of advanced mammary cancer. Ibid., *146:*471, 1951.
Pearson, O. H., Eliel, L. P., Rawson, R. W., Dobriner, K., and Rhoads, C. P.: ACTH and cortisone-induced regression of lymphoid tumors. Cancer, *2:*943, 1949.
Savlov, E. D., and Schilling, J. A.: Cancer of the male breast treated by orchiectomy. Surgery, *28:*867, 1950.
Sprague, R. G., Mason, H. L., and Power, M. H.: Physiologic effects of cortisone and ACTH in man. Recent Progr. Hormone Research, *6:*315, 1951.
Thorn, G. W., and Forsham, P. H.: Adrenal cortical insufficiency; in Williams, R. H.: Textbook of Endocrinology. Philadelphia, W. B. Saunders Company, 1950, p. 248.
———, Forsham, P. H., Frawley, T. F., Wilson, D. L., Renold, A. E., Fredrickson, D. S., and Jenkins, D.: Advances in the diagnosis and treatment of adrenal insufficiency. Am. J. Med., *10:*595, 1951.
Twombly, G. H.: The relation of hormones to testicular tumors; in Endocrinology of Neoplastic Diseases. New York, Oxford University Press, 1947, p. 242.

CHAPTER 7

THE THYROID GLAND

ANATOMY AND EMBRYOLOGY

The thyroid gland develops as an invagination of the floor of the embryonic pharynx. This process descends as a cellular stalk to the anterior

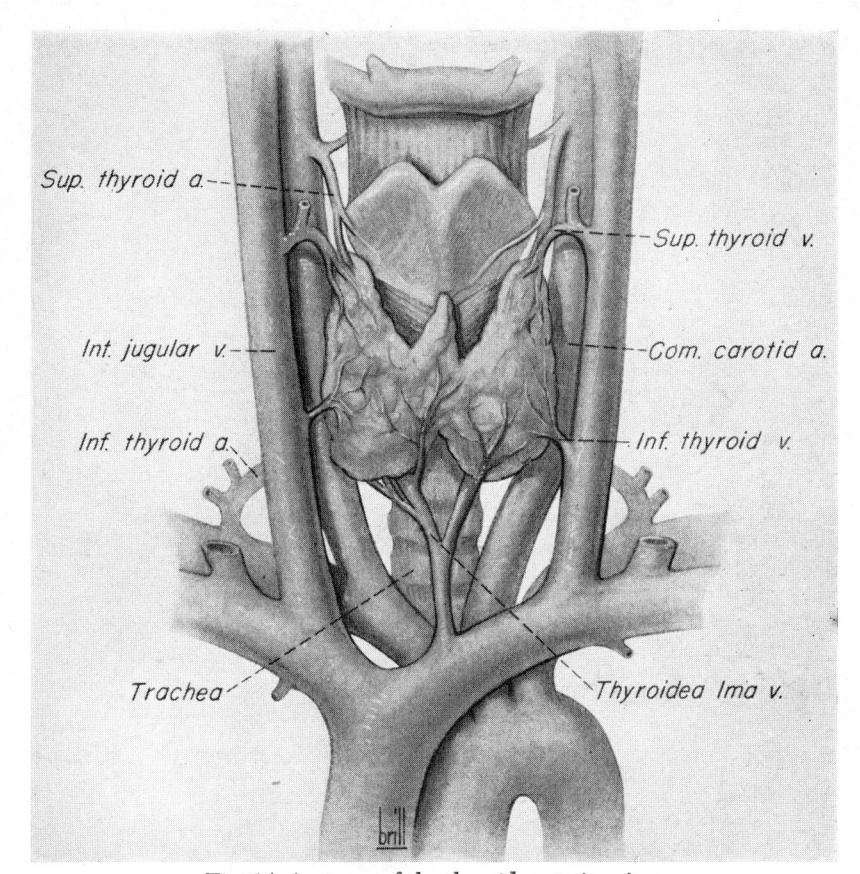

Fig. 14. Anatomy of the thyroid, anterior view.

part of the neck and then by proliferation of its cells gives rise to the epithelial elements which are later to become the adult organ. The connection with the pharynx, known as the thyroglossal tract, usually dis-

70   SURGERY AND THE ENDOCRINE SYSTEM

appears and is represented only by the foramen caecum on the back of the tongue. If this process does persist, it may give rise to the familiar thyroglossal cyst.

The normal thyroid consists of two lateral lobes approximately equal in size which are connected in the middle across the ventral surface of

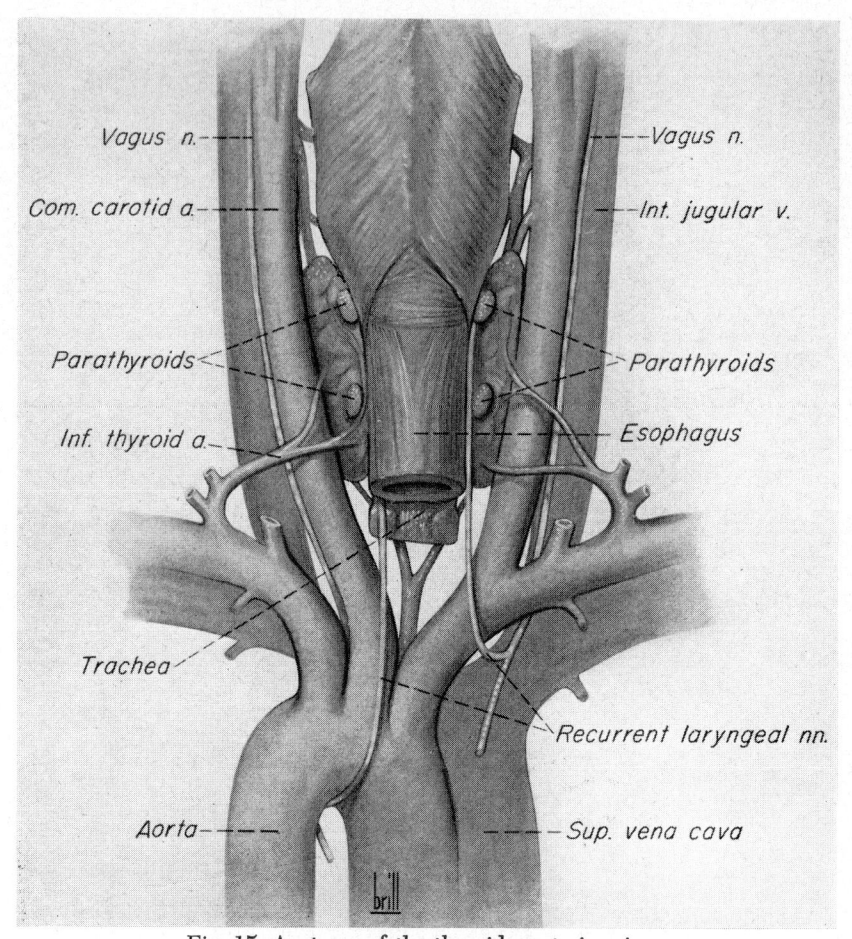

Fig. 15. Anatomy of the thyroid, posterior view.

the trachea by a band of thyroid tissue called the isthmus. Extending cephalad from the isthmus may be still another projection of thyroid tissue, the pyramidal lobe. The gland is attached to the front and lateral aspects of the larynx and upper trachea and extends from the thyroid cartilage downward to the fourth or fifth tracheal ring. Usually the isthmus overlies the second and third tracheal rings. Overlying the thyroid from front to back are the skin, superficial fascia, platysma muscle, deep cervical fascia, sternothyroid muscles, sternohyoid muscles, and the inner borders of the sternocleidomastoid muscles. Lateral and pos-

THE THYROID GLAND

terior on each side is the carotid sheath enclosing the vagus nerve, carotid artery and internal jugular vein. The thyroid itself is enclosed in a thin adherent capsule which posteriorly is attached to the trachea. Identification of this capsule is vital if technical errors are to be consistently avoided.

The arterial blood supply to the thyroid gland is derived principally from the paired superior and inferior thyroid arteries arising from the external carotid and thyrocervical axis, respectively. There is often a small artery to the isthmus from above, and the thyroidea ima may arise from the aorta below and terminate in the isthmus.

The venous drainage of the thyroid is extensive. The superior thyroid vein accompanies the superior thyroid artery and passes over the common carotid artery to empty into either the internal jugular vein or the lingual vein. The middle or lateral thyroid vein, an important operative landmark on either side, empties into the lower part of the internal jugular vein. Finally, communicating freely with the superior and middle thyroid veins after arising from the plexus on the surface of the gland, the several inferior thyroid veins drain usually into the right and left innominate veins, though occasionally they may empty into the subclavian or internal jugular vein.

The recurrent laryngeal nerves are branches of the vagus nerves. The right nerve passes behind the subclavian artery, and the left nerve curves around the aorta. They then ascend on either side, crossing in front, behind, or between the branches of the inferior thyroid arteries and run beneath the lateral lobes of the thyroid closely adjacent to the trachea until they enter the larynx to supply most of the intrinsic muscles except the cricothyroid.

The parathyroids, usually four in number, are brownish red in color and resemble small lymph nodes 6 to 7 mm. long, 3 to 4 mm. broad, and about 2 mm. thick. The location of the two upper parathyroids on the posterior capsule near each upper pole is fairly constant. The lower parathyroids are far more variable in position and, while most often on the posterior surface near each lower pole, may be found lower in the neck or in the mediastinum. Rarely one or more parathyroids may be situated within the thyroid tissue.

PHYSIOLOGY OF THE THYROID GLAND

As far as is presently known, the physiologic action of the thyroid gland is dependent entirely upon the effects of thyroxine. Many fea-

$$HO-\underset{I}{\overset{I}{\bigcirc}}-O-\underset{I}{\overset{I}{\bigcirc}}-CH_2CH\underset{COOH}{\overset{NH_2}{\diagup}}$$

Thyroxine

tures of thyroid physiology have been touched upon in previous chapters and this discussion will be limited to a brief review of the clinical effects of the thyroid hormone. The following list of activities is taken from Means (with additions):

1. Calorigenic action (basal metabolic rate).
2. Action upon the growth, maturation and differentiation of tissue (cretinism).
3. Action upon body water, salts and proteins (abnormal fluid and protein deposits in myxedema).
4. Action upon carbohydrate metabolism (glycosuria and deranged glucose tolerance in hyperthyroidism).
5. Action on lipids (increased serum cholesterol in hypothyroidism).
6. Action upon the nervous system (increased irritability).
7. Action upon the muscular system (may be associated with, or independent of, effects on nervous system; manifested by myasthenia and, in severe cases, muscular atrophy).
8. Action upon the circulatory system. This action is in part secondary to the increased circulation resulting from the effects above; however, Leblond and Hoff and Hoffman, Hoffman and Talesnik have demonstrated a direct effect of thyroxine on the heart (Chapter 1).

PATHOLOGY OF THE THYROID GLAND
Nontoxic Goiter

Nontoxic Diffuse (Colloid, Endemic) Goiter. This is characterized grossly by a diffuse symmetric enlargement of the thyroid gland and microscopically by a flattening of the follicular epithelium and distention of the acini with excessive amounts of colloid. Such glands may reach an enormous size. While there may be other contributing factors, the most common single *etiology* is an absolute lack of iodine, and prophylaxis by the administration of iodine is thus important in goitrous regions.

Treatment. The treatment of the established condition depends upon the age of the patient and the size and position of the gland. Endemic goiter still in the hyperplastic stage should disappear upon the ingestion of iodine, but after the colloid stage has been reached this therapy is of limited value (Means). Desiccated thyroid in moderate doses may at times cause regression of such goiters and improve the general condition of the patient, particularly if the moderate hypothyroidism which often accompanies this disease is present.

Surgical treatment may be indicated merely because of the size of the gland. Pressure from these goiters may result in dysphagia, dysphonia or dyspnea, and the mass may effect considerable disfigurement. In addition, they may later become nodular with the inherent possibility of malignant degeneration or the development of toxicity. For these reasons, the writer believes that large endemic goiters which do not regress under medical treatment should be removed surgically.

THE THYROID GLAND

Nontoxic Nodular Goiter* (**Adenomatous Goiter without Hyperthyroidism**). This is most frequent in the geographic areas where colloid goiter is endemic. Here also a deficiency of iodine may be foremost among the etiologic possibilities. As noted above, a diffuse colloid goiter may, in involution, become nodular. Adenomatous masses of the thyroid may be single or multiple, and they may involve only one lobe or both lobes. For descriptive purposes we have termed the diffuse enlargement of only one lobe a "nodular goiter." Frequently a single adenoma deep

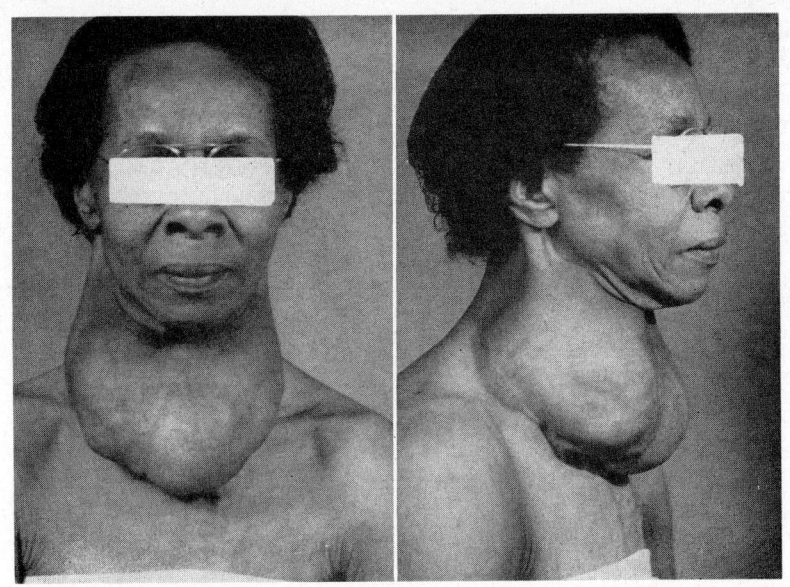

Fig. 16. Large nontoxic nodular goiter. This gland was readily movable and was easily resected.

within the thyroid substance is completely or partially encapsulated and when exposed "shells out" quite readily. Again, there may be many nodular masses. The microscopic picture may be extremely varied, some nodules presenting hemorrhage, others regions of degeneration and even calcification, and still others hypertrophic changes in the follicles. Occasionally a fetal type of thyroid tissue may be seen.

Clinical Considerations. From the extremely varied type of microscopic pictures found in different adenomas it is readily appreciated that various complications of nontoxic nodular goiter may be anticipated. Among these are hemorrhage into a follicle with sudden pressure symptoms, gradual pressure symptoms from a slowly growing cervical or intrathoracic mass, development of toxicity, cosmetic defects and, most important, the possibility of malignant degeneration.

* A goiter is considered nodular unless it presents a diffuse enlargement of both lobes. A smooth adenomatous enlargement of only one lobe is considered a nodular goiter.

Treatment. The treatment of choice is surgical resection. The morbidity and mortality for this operation in competent hands is exceedingly small, and against this low mortality one must weigh the strong possibility of future complications, of which cancer is the most serious. The reported incidence of malignancy ranges from 5 to 20 per cent in different clinics. Lahey and Hare have recently reported an incidence of 10 per cent in solitary nodules. At the Hospital of the University of Pennsylvania, the incidence of carcinoma in all goiters removed at operation, exclusive of toxic glands, has been 9.2 per cent over the past six years (Horn). Hinton and Lord reported a 6.7 per cent incidence of carcinoma

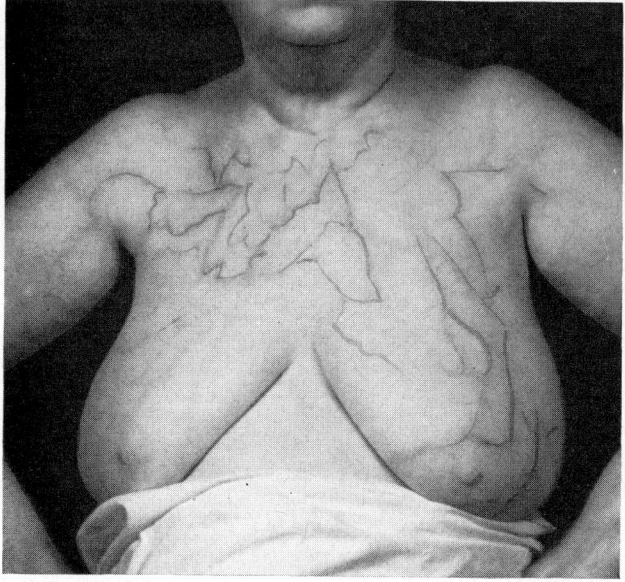

Fig. 17. Infrared photograph of distended veins in patient with large intrathoracic goiter.

in seventy-five consecutive breast nodules and a 7.6 per cent incidence of carcinoma in 184 thyroid nodules. Crile reports an incidence of carcinoma of 10.9 per cent in surgically removed nontoxic nodular goiters and 24.5 per cent in surgically removed nontoxic solitary tumors of the thyroid. However, he is careful to point out that the discrepancy between the high incidence of cancer of the thyroid encountered by surgeons (Cole) and the low incidence of fatal cancer of the thyroid reported in vital statistics (Rogers and associates) likely reflects a progressive screening of patients who finally come to operation. There are many small (less than 2.5 cm. diameter) soft nodules which disappear while under observation by the patient himself or by the internist. However, the hard solitary nodule should be removed, for it is a lesion of this type that is most frequently the site of cancer. Finally, since statistics can only indicate chance as it affects a large group, the particular goiter under consideration is to be dealt with on the basis of whether or not surgery or watchful waiting seems to be to the best interest of that particular patient.

Hyperthyroidism

Toxic Nodular Goiter; Toxic Diffuse Goiter (Graves' Disease, Exophthalmic Goiter)

Etiology. The fundamental pathogenesis of hyperthyroidism remains unknown. Recent studies by Heinbecker and others have indicated the presence of neural pathways through which the higher cerebral centers may stimulate the anterior pituitary to secrete excessive amounts of the thyroid stimulating hormone; studies of this type are of especial interest in view of the frequency with which states of increased thyroid activity follow hard on the heels of situations of severe emotional stress. Nevertheless, such relationships have not been fully established. What is certain is that most of the clinical signs and symptoms of thyrotoxicosis result from an increased production of thyroxine. The diagnosis and treatment of the disease are based upon this fact.

Signs and Symptoms. The physical findings and symptomatology of thyrotoxicosis result from increased thyroxine effects. An increased calorigenic action causes a sensation of warmth, sweating, moist skin, peripheral dilatation and weight loss associated with a voracious appetite. Circulatory effects cause tachycardia, increased pulse pressure, increased cardiac irritability, increased cardiac output and ultimate cardiac decompensation. The nervous and muscular findings are an increased irritability, excessive activity, intoxication and occasional psychosis, tremor, palpitation, diarrhea, myasthenia and muscular atrophy. There is an excessive fluid turnover, and oligomenorrhea or amenorrhea may occur in females. Patients with toxic diffuse goiter are particularly likely to present some degree of exophthalmus. This finding is thought to be due to a pituitary hormone and not to an increased amount of thyroxine per se, since the proptosis may occur in the absence of hyperthyroidism and vice versa.

When most of these findings are present in a given case a qualitative diagnosis of hyperthyroidism is readily made. However, the majority of patients with this disease have only moderate degrees of thyroid overactivity and hence may easily pass undiagnosed unless the clinician keeps hyperthyroidism high on his list of causes of fatigue, weight loss, mild tachycardia, amenorrhea or sterility. Even when suspected, hyperthyroidism may prove to be an exceedingly difficult diagnosis to make clinically.

The Laboratory Diagnosis of Hyperthyroidism. The tests currently considered the most useful are the following:

1. The basal metabolic rate (BMR) (normal range, -15 to $+15$ per cent)

2. The serum level of protein bound iodine (PBI) (normal range, 3 to 6 gamma per 100 ml. of serum)
3. The uptake of radioiodine by the thyroid gland (normal range, 10 to 40 per cent)
4. The conversion ratio (normal range, 10 to 45 per cent)

The Basal Metabolic Rate. Although the BMR is the most widely used of these tests, it is not the most reliable measure of thyroid activity available. Even when technical imperfections in the performance of the test have been excluded, the patient may find it impossible to achieve a truly basal condition. Benedict has shown that an emotional disturbance may cause a marked increase in the BMR which may not subside for several days. The test can be performed under pentothal anesthesia, but this is often not advisable. A repeatedly normal BMR will rule out hyperthyroidism in all but the very exceptional case, but a persistently elevated rate does not necessarily mean that the patient has thyroid overactivity. There are other conditions which may be associated with an increase in the basal metabolic rate, and among these are pheochromocytoma, acromegaly, leukemia, essential hypertension, certain drugs, pregnancy, infections, fever, polycythemia vera and the administration of thyroid extract. Needless to say, in cardiac failure or in any type of respiratory obstruction the BMR determination is unreliable. Since at times it may be impossible to exclude all these conditions, this test has definite limitations.

Protein-Bound Iodine Level of Serum. The organic fraction of the serum iodine has been shown to bear a dependable direct relationship to the degree of thyroid activity, and this fraction is now considered to represent the quantitative measurement of the iodine of thyroxine and related compounds circulating in the blood stream. A carefully performed serum protein-bound iodine determination is an accurate measurement of the level of thyroid activity, provided the patient has not recently received iodine compounds or thyroid extract. The ingestion of iodine in any form renders the test suspect for some time; as an extreme example, Man and Peters have shown that the instillation of lipiodol for bronchography may cause a spurious elevation of the serum PBI level for as long as fifteen months. However, with adequate precautions this test, though laborious, is superior to the BMR in that it is a more objective determination and is not affected by most of the numerous conditions which render the BMR unreliable. The serum PBI level is not affected by thiouracil administration. We have found the normal range of the serum PBI level to lie between 3 and 6 micrograms per 100 ml. of serum, and this agrees well with results obtained by other laboratories using the same method. Values above this range indicate thyrotoxicosis and values below this range indicate a state of hypothyroidism. If the serum PBI level is within normal limits the patient almost certainly does not have thyrotoxicosis; however, this cannot

THE THYROID GLAND

be said for the BMR, since an increase in thyroid activity of thirty points (from −15 to +15) might have taken place shortly preceding a test which showed a BMR of +15.

Uptake of Radioactive Iodine by the Thyroid Gland. The availability of the radioactive isotope of iodine has made it possible to employ the avidity of the thyroid gland for elemental iodine as a measure of thyroid activity. Hertz, Roberts and Salter demonstrated a direct correlation between the functional state of this organ and the amount of radioactive iodine stored there over a definite period of time. The normal range of uptake in man was found to be between 10 and 40 per cent. An uptake in excess of 50 per cent was held to be specific for thyroid hyperactivity,

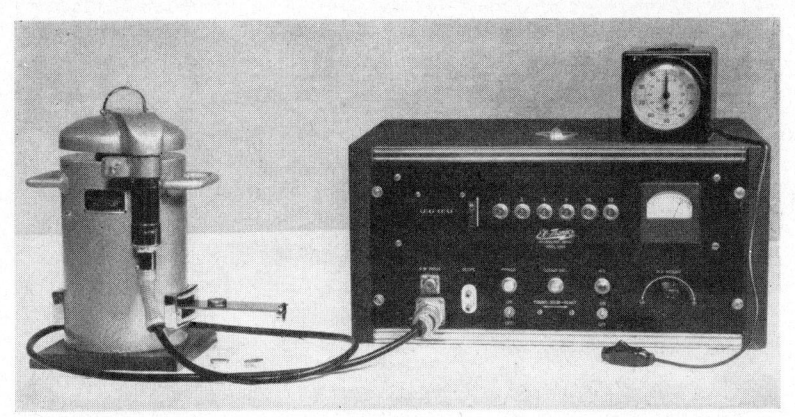

Fig. 18. Radioactivity counting equipment. This apparatus is easily handled and may be used for performing conversion ratios with radioiodine or for determining potassium and sodium pools using radioisotopes of these elements. (Courtesy of Dr. Richard H. Chamberlain and The Department of Radiology, Hospital of the University of Pennsylvania.)

though there was a slight overlap between the euthyroid and hyperthyroid patients. This additional test of thyroid function is now employed extensively in the larger clinical centers and has proved an exceedingly valuable tool in the investigation of thyroid physiology.

Aside from the fairly expensive equipment required for the safe clinical use of radioiodine, this test has the following disadvantages: It is unreliable if the patient has recently received thiouracil compounds or iodine therapy; factitial thyrotoxicosis resulting from uncontrolled oral therapy with desiccated thyroid for such conditions as sterility would not be detected by a measure of the activity of the thyroid gland; and the uptake of radioactive iodine in goiters which are partially or wholly intrathoracic often cannot be determined accurately.

Conversion Ratio. In a series of investigations employing radioiodine as a tracer in the study of thyroid physiology, Chaikoff, Taurog and Reinhardt found that the rate of incorporation of radioactive iodine into protein by the thyroid was increased in rats and guinea pigs injected with thyrotropic hormone. These workers suggested that the rate of conversion of radioactive iodine into thyroxine might be used to measure thyroid activity. Subsequently Clark, Moe and Adams found that in man the conversion ratio ranged from 13 to 40 per cent. Those patients whose conversion ratio was 50 per cent or greater were considered to have thyroid hyperactivity, and in a study of 150 patients we have obtained similar results. If the conversion ratio has a definite advantage over the thyroid uptake of radioactive iodine as a measure of thyroid activity, it perhaps lies in the fact that presumably the conversion ratio measures the actual rate of thyroxine formation and is not affected by the anatomic location of the thyroid tissue.

General Discussion of Tests for the Diagnosis of Hyperthyroidism. It should not be concluded that any one test of thyroid activity should be used to the exclusion of all others. On the contrary, since each of the four tests discussed above measures a different facet of thyroid physiology the tests supplement one another, and in certain situations all may be useful. For example, thyrotoxicosis associated with an intrathoracic goiter might not be accurately measured by the iodine uptake because of the goiter's anatomic location. The BMR could be erroneous due to pressure on the respiratory tract. The serum protein-bound iodine level would be elevated, but the conversion ratio would be required to distinguish between factitial thyrotoxicosis and true hyperactivity of the intrathoracic goiter. We have reported such a case in which thyrotoxicosis was indeed factitial and was not due to hyperactivity of the patient's huge intrathoracic goiter. Thyroid hyperactivity in patients who have received thiouracil compounds is best diagnosed by determination of the BMR and serum PBI level, since even small amounts of these drugs modify the uptake of iodine by the thyroid gland. The recent ingestion of iodine compounds tends to render suspect the serum PBI level, the conversion ratio and the radioiodine uptake by the thyroid gland. Thus, iodine therapy should be avoided until a quantitative diagnosis of the level of thyroid activity has been made. Finally, at times a combination of circumstances may render all the laboratory tests unreliable, and under these circumstances a clinical trial of iodine therapy may prove useful.

The Management of Toxic Goiter

While taking cognizance of the fact that toxic nodular goiter and toxic diffuse goiter (Graves' disease) may present quite contrasting clinical pictures and that their fundamental etiology may also be different, the general therapeutic objective of all types of treatment for hyperthyroidism is the same, namely, the reduction of the level of thyroxine available to the body tissues. In this way a satisfactory therapeutic result may be obtained in the absence of factual knowledge as to the mechanism by which the thyroid is stimulated to produce excessive amounts of its hor-

THE THYROID GLAND

mone. The therapeutic methods by which the activity of this target organ, the thyroid, is altered are simple iodine therapy, thiouracil compounds, roentgen irradiation, radioactive iodine and subtotal thyroidectomy. So far as definitive therapy is concerned, we will consider the first three of these measures in a few sentences and devote the remainder of the discussion to a consideration of the last two.

Simple inorganic iodine is not the treatment of choice for primary hyperthyroidism. It may at times have a place in effecting a remission of mild recurrent hyperthyroidism as a means of averting further surgery, but even here radioactive iodine may prove to be more reliable. Thio-

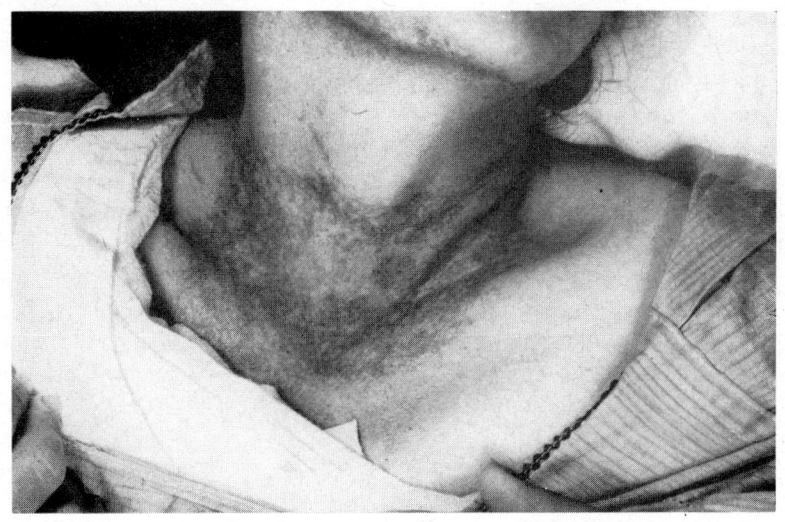

Fig. 19. Skin changes secondary to roentgen therapy.

uracil, propylthiouracil, and similar compounds have been effective in producing permanent remissions in some cases of mild thyrotoxicosis, particularly in diffuse goiters. However, the frequency of recurrence following cessation of treatment, the time and expense involved in the control of this therapy, and the distinct possibility of carcinogenesis following prolonged stimulation of the thyroid by these goitrogenic compounds have made it apparent that for the time being these drugs have their greatest value in the preparation of the patient for safe subtotal thyroidectomy. External roentgen therapy over the thyroid gland, formerly recommended in certain patients considered poor operative risks, will likely be replaced by internal irradiation in the form of orally administered radioiodine.

General Considerations in the Choice Between Subtotal Thyroidectomy and Radioactive Iodine as a Means of Therapy for Toxic Goiter. Since the early work of Hertz and Roberts and of Hamilton and Soley with radioiodine as a means of therapy in hyperthyroidism, this type of treatment has been fairly well standardized through the efforts of numerous investigators. Sufficient time has now elapsed to permit certain preliminary conclusions. Beyond question, radioactive iodine will reduce thyroid activity and even produce myxedema in practically every patient, if sufficient dosage is given. This material, with or without carrier, can be administered in a glass of water, and such convenient therapy has a very real appeal to both patient and practitioner, especially in comparison with subtotal thyroidectomy. However, a very large segment of opinion still regards radioiodine therapy as experimental and prefers to bear in mind the following possible sequelae of such treatment when planning the management of the individual thyrotoxic patient. First, as is now well known, malignancy induced by prolonged, low-grade irradiation may not appear for from ten to twenty years. While the half-life of I^{131} is such that most of its energy is released in thirty days, some question concerning its carcinogenic effect is likely to persist for years. Second, in young women the possible effect of radioactive iodine on the ovaries, especially as regards the mutation of chromosomes of primordial ova, must be considered. Third, the relatively poor response of toxic nodular goiter, as compared with toxic diffuse goiter, to radioactive iodine therapy must be weighed against the possibility of subsequent development of carcinoma in any nodular goiter. In most uncomplicated cases of toxic nodular goiter we consider subtotal thyroidectomy definitely the treatment of choice at the present time. The general situations which may be considered appropriate for each of these two types of therapy are as follows:

SUBTOTAL THYROIDECTOMY	RADIOACTIVE IODINE
Uncomplicated toxic diffuse goiter in the young, particularly in women	Intolerance to antithyroid drugs
	Hyperthyroidism refractory to drug therapy
Toxic nodular goiter	Thyrocardiac disease
	Recurrent postoperative hyperthyroidism
	Severe exophthalmus
	Poor operative risks with either toxic nodular or toxic diffuse goiter

If the listed theoretic objections to the use of radioactive iodine are convincingly removed during the next few years, this agent will become the treatment of choice for practically all toxic diffuse goiters whose size does not preclude a satisfactory cosmetic result. Also, further knowledge and refinements may render radioiodine therapy still more effective in the treatment of toxic nodular goiter.

Radioactive Iodine Therapy in Hyperthyroidism. The treatment of hyperthyroidism with radioactive iodine is exceedingly simple. By means of a preliminary "tracer dose" of approximately 200 microcuries of radioiodine given by mouth, the uptake of radioiodine by the thyroid gland is measured to gain some idea of the degree of excessive activity present. The size of the gland is also estimated by physical examination. Using the rate of function and the size of the gland, the probable dosage of radioiodine required is then estimated. Chapman and Evans advise the oral administration of a total dose of from 6 to 10 millicuries in a single drink such as water for the average goitrous patient. Although it may be necessary to repeat the dosage when small amounts are administered initially, this method of treatment would seem far safer than to risk permanent myxedema and excessive irradiation of the thyroid, larynx and possibly other tissues by using large initial doses. The patient should then be re-examined at monthly intervals, since the full effect of a single dose of radioiodine may not become apparent for several months.

Subtotal Thyroidectomy. *Preoperative Preparation.* The successful treatment of hyperthyroid states by subtotal thyroidectomy encompasses far more than mere operative intervention. It implies the careful preparation of the patient for surgery, proper selection of anesthesia, skillful surgical technic and judgment, and continued care postoperatively until the patient is safely past the possible complications.

SPECIFIC THYROID THERAPY. Even before the advent of thiouracil compounds, the preoperative use of iodine therapy as championed by Plummer in 1922 had greatly reduced the hazards of thyroidectomy, particularly with respect to the dreaded postoperative crisis. Following the demonstration in 1943 by Astwood and his associates that the administration of certain sulfonamides or thiourea to normal rats resulted in an enlarged, hyperemic and hyperplastic thyroid accompanied by a state of hypothyroidism, other similar compounds were tried and found to be even more successful in the suppression of excessive thyroid activity in human beings. Of these compounds, thiouracil and propylthiouracil have been the most widely used. The use of thiouracil has been gradually abandoned because of its toxicity, but propylthiouracil has proved extremely valuable in bringing the BMR to within normal limits and thus permitting subtotal thyroidectomy on an essentially euthyroid patient. An effective dosage regimen consists of the oral administration of 100 mg. three times a day for as long as necessary to bring the BMR to within normal limits. This usually requires several weeks. These goitrogenic compounds increase the vascularity of the gland and make thyroidectomy more difficult, and for this reason many surgeons prefer to administer iodine during the last week before operation, with or without propylthiouracil.

THERAPEUTIC ADJUNCTS. The presence of prolonged thyrotoxicosis usually results in a state of depleted nutritional reserves accompanied by the derangements in the physiologic response to trauma outlined in the chapter on nutrition. Fatty infiltration in the liver should be minimized by a sound dietary policy while the patient is receiving antithyroid preparation. Liberal amounts of proteins, calories and vitamins

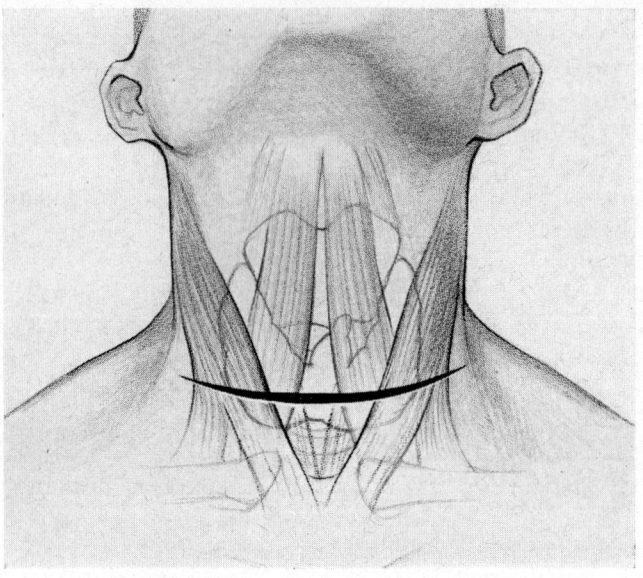

Fig. 20. Incision for thyroidectomy.

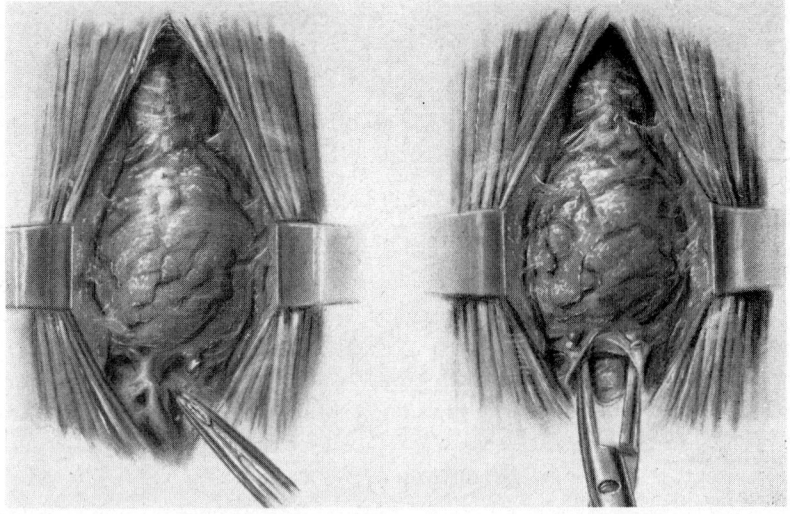

Fig. 21. Subtotal thyroidectomy. After the gland has been adequately exposed with or without division of the strap muscles, we prefer to divide the isthmus as a first step. *Left:* The hemostat is shown grasping the divided branch of the inferior thyroid vein, a guide to the position of the trachea. The fellow vein to the left is undivided. *Right:* The initial step is the exposure of the trachea with a stock hemostat. (Johnson, J.: Ann. Surg. 99:697, 1934; J. B. Lippincott Company.)

should be supplied. Sedation is given for the hyperirritable neuromuscular system, and the patient is humored when he makes what could

THE THYROID GLAND

be considered unreasonable requests. Such excessive attitudes on the part of the patient usually disappear when his disease is controlled.

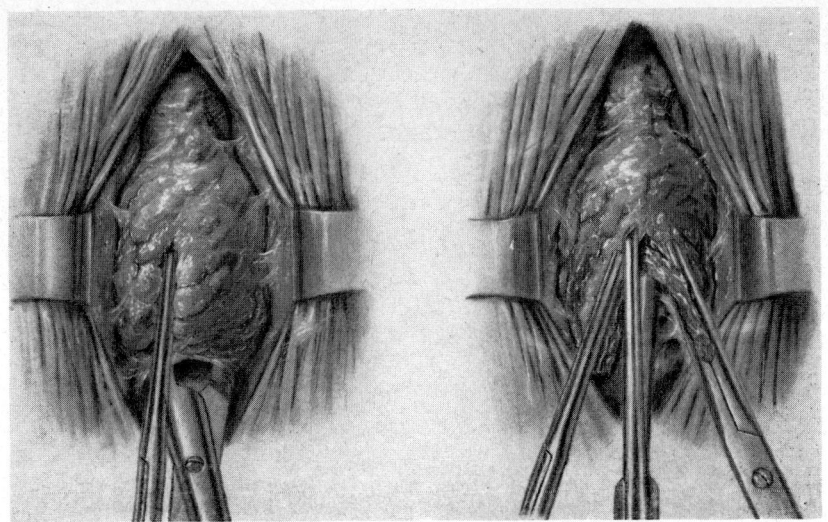

Fig. 22. Subtotal thyroidectomy. *Left:* The isthmus is shown separated from the trachea; a Kocher hemostat has been applied. *Right:* Two Kocher hemostats have been applied to the first section of the isthmus with division of same. (Johnson, J.: Ann. Surg., 99:697, 1934; J. B. Lippincott Company.)

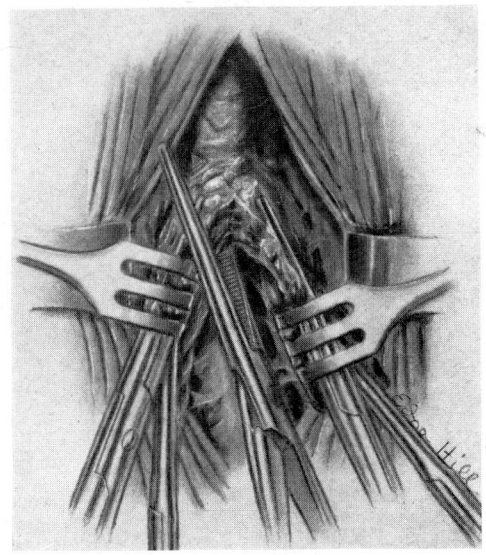

Fig. 23. Subtotal thyroidectomy. Division of isthmus continued, section by section. Only a small portion remains. (Johnson, J.: Ann. Surg., 99:698, 1934; J. B. Lippincott Company.)

The cardiovascular system is evaluated, and the patient is digitalized if the internist finds it advisable.

ANESTHESIA FOR THYROIDECTOMY. The individual surgeon is likely to have his own personal preference as to anesthesia. This results from the fact that in his hands a particular type of anesthesia has given the most satisfactory results. We have found local infiltration or cervical block with procaine following basal sedation with morphine sulfate and/or a

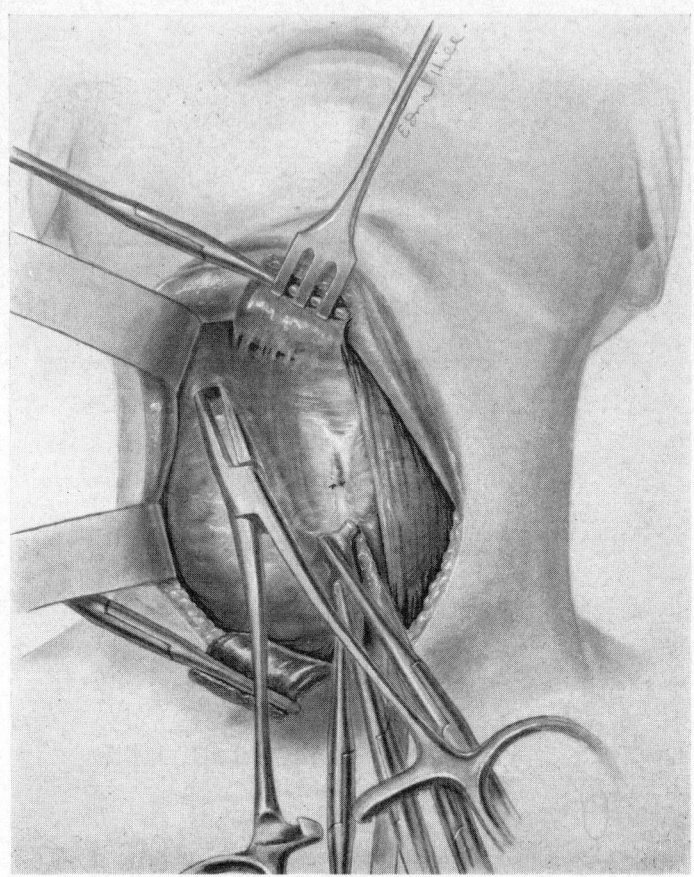

Fig. 24. Subtotal thyroidectomy. Diagrammatic sketch showing approach to structures of upper pole. (Frazier, C. H., and Erb, W.: Ann. Surg., *101*:1353, 1935; J. B. Lippincott Company.)

barbiturate a very successful anesthetic in patients who are poor operative risks, whose gland is not too large, or whose recurrent nerve on one side has been previously damaged. However, most patients do not care to be awake throughout operations so closely adjacent to the sense organs, and in the presence of large glands such anesthesia is likely to be inadequate. We most frequently use a general anesthetic mixture containing oxygen and one or all of the following: nitrous oxide, ether and cyclopropane. When considered advisable, the anesthetic is administered through an endotracheal tube.

THE THYROID GLAND

Operative Technic: Safeguards, Complications, and Their Management. The detailed technic of this anatomic dissection will be found in the accompanying illustrations and in appropriate manuals. We shall confine these comments to a consideration of some of the difficulties which may be encountered with thyroidectomy.

In any successful undertaking the magnitude of the task and the possible difficulties which may arise are first measured objectively. A small

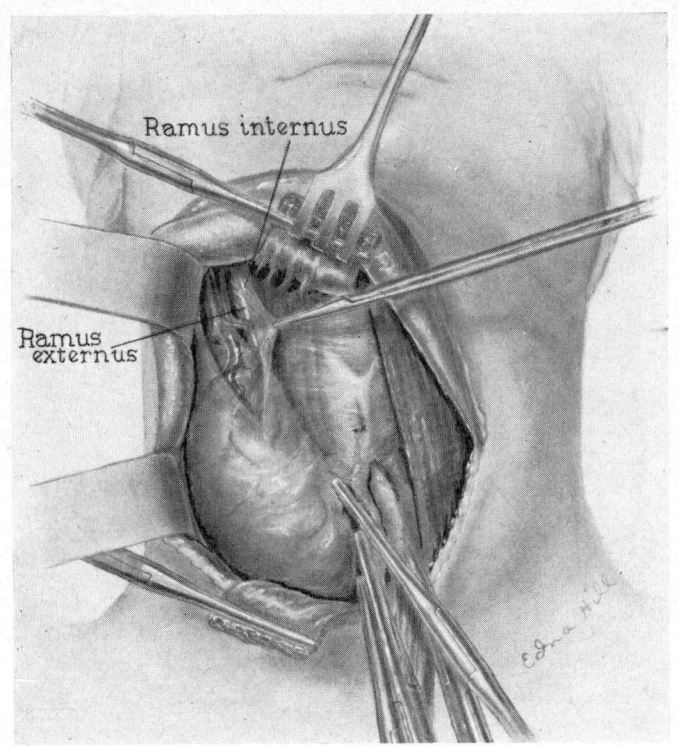

Fig. 25. Subtotal thyroidectomy. Exposure of superior pole vessels and superior laryngeal nerve. (Frazier, C. H., and Erb, W.: Ann. Surg., *101*:1353, 1935; J. B. Lippincott Company.)

goiter is usually removed easily and there are few complications. However, a total thyroidectomy on any gland, or a subtotal thyroidectomy on a large gland, may prove difficult. A toxic gland is likely to be more vascular and more friable than a nontoxic gland. A preoperative chest roentgenogram to determine whether or not the gland extends into the upper mediastinum is frequently helpful. Calcification in a hard gland makes it somewhat less likely that the gland harbors malignancy.

TIME FOR OPERATION. The surgeon must himself judge when the patient is ready for operation. If the BMR has declined to within normal limits and remains there, if the pulse rate has declined and stabilized, if the patient has gained even a few pounds, and if the rest of the clinical picture is satisfactory, then the operation can usually be performed with safety.

BLOOD LOSS. The amount of blood lost at a given thyroidectomy varies enormously depending upon whether or not the gland has been toxic, whether or not it is the site of inflammation, and whether or not malignancy is present. In glands of excessive size it is well to be prepared with a 15-gauge needle in the vein and blood on hand in the operating

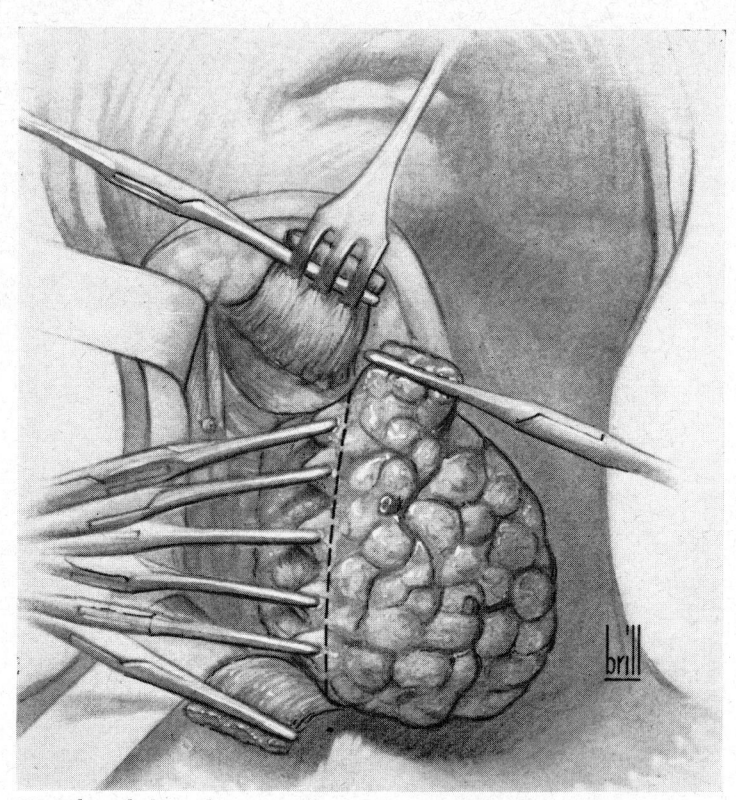

Fig. 26. Subtotal thyroidectomy. The superior pole has been divided, and the lobe has been reflected upward and medially. The ring of hemostats serves to delineate the remnant of the lobe which is to be preserved. The next step is to excise the remainder of the lobe.

room. By dividing the isthmus as a first step, the operator can more easily control bleeding if a large vessel is inadvertently torn.

CARDIAC ARREST AND VENTRICULAR FIBRILLATION. This condition may be no more frequent in thyroid operations than in other procedures, exclusive of operations involving the chest, but the author has been associated with several such episodes in thyroid patients. As emphasized by Johnson and Kirby, when the pulse is suddenly no longer discernible and there has not been excessive blood loss, one must not hesitate to enter the left side of the thorax through the left fourth or fifth interspace an-

THE THYROID GLAND

teriorly and massage the heart. This is often sufficient stimulus to cause the heart to resume its beat immediately. However, we have seen a heart resume beating as late as forty-five minutes after the beginning of massage. If ventricular fibrillation is present, the heart should be shocked with an electric current. Simultaneously with the massage, the anesthetist should continue to inflate the lungs with a mixture high in oxygen and the rapid infusion of blood under pressure should be maintained.

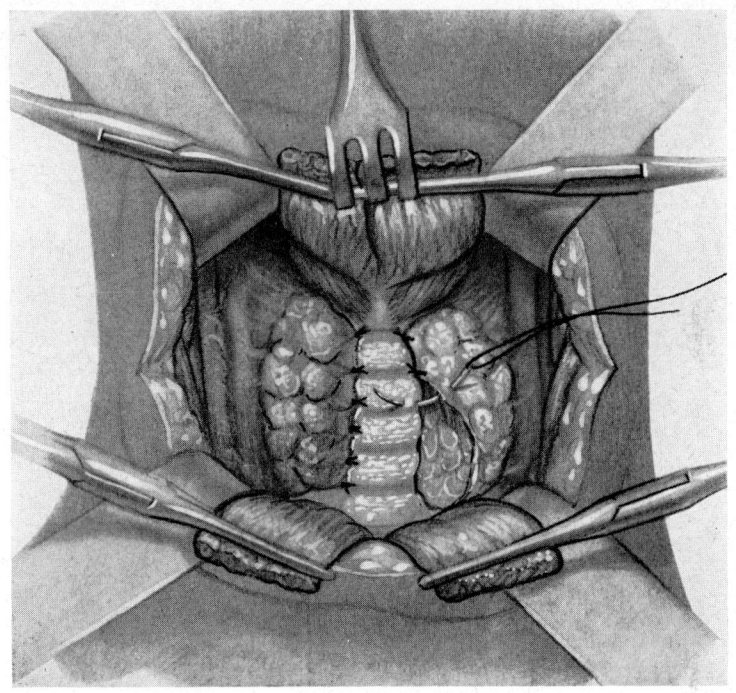

Fig. 27. Subtotal thyroidectomy. Hemostatic sutures are shown gently but snugly joining the capsule of the remnant of each lobe to the pretracheal fascia. The writer prefers to use fine catgut throughout with the single exception of silk or cotton for closure of the skin. Eighty to ninety per cent of the toxic gland is resected.

By such prompt and vigorous measures Johnson and Kirby have saved eight of their last twelve cases of cardiac arrest.

FATAL AIR EMBOLISM. This is a complication of thyroidectomy which is much less frequent than the emphasis placed upon it in the literature would lead one to suppose. Though the writer has never encountered such an instance, care should of course be taken to prevent air from entering large veins.

RECURRENT NERVES. There are two schools of thought concerning the operative management of the recurrent laryngeal nerves. One school advises that the nerves be routinely exposed, while the other holds that the operator should "know where the nerves are and avoid them." It seems inescapable, however, that as more radical thyroid surgery is performed for cancer the surgeon must deliberately identify and preserve these nerves. It is our practice to examine the cords preoperatively and immediately postoperatively. If the patient then becomes hoarse after the cords have moved normally immediately following operation, one can suspect inflammatory edema and predict that normal motility of the cords will probably be restored. Where there is reason to feel that the nerve has been injured in doing a particularly radical resection on one side, it is well to allow the patient to wake up and to examine the cords before proceeding to do an equally radical resection on the second side. If this is not done, the greatest care should be exercised on the

TABLE 10

Management of Cardiac Arrest

1. Prompt and bold action is essential.
2. If the pulse and blood pressure are suddenly no longer obtainable and excessive blood loss has not occurred, immediately open the left side of the thorax through the fourth or fifth interspace anteriorly and massage the heart at a rate of from 60 to 120 squeezes per minute.
3. Simultaneously, begin a rapid intravenous infusion of fluid (blood preferred) under pressure.
4. Inflate lungs with a respirator, an anesthetist's bag or, if no other method is available, by the mouth-to-mouth technic.
5. If it is noted that the ventricles are fibrillating, the heart should be shocked with an electric current to stop the fibrillation and permit the normal rhythm to take over.
6. Hearts have resumed normal rhythm after even 45 minutes of massage.

second side and, unless absolutely necessary, a less radical resection should be carried out.

PARATHYROIDS. There has been the same divergence of opinion concerning whether or not the parathyroids should be routinely identified and preserved by direct visualization, or whether they should be preserved by keeping the dissection within the thyroid capsule. While the latter course is successful in most cases, it cannot be used where complete resection of the thyroid is indicated. Moreover, in the surgery of the parathyroids themselves, the exposure and identification of these glands is essential. Thus, while most thyroid resections can be done safely without exposing the parathyroid glands, the surgeon must be able to recognize these structures readily when this is required.

If the patient shows signs of tetany postoperatively, a considered plan of management should be instituted. First, a blood specimen for determinations of serum calcium (normal value 10 ±1 mg.) and phosphorus (normal value 3.5 ±0.5 mg.) should be drawn. At the same time 10 to 20 cc. of 10 per cent calcium gluconate may be given intravenously; this usually results in immediate relaxation of the spasm. However, since the effect of this medication is brief, one should at once administer large doses of calcium lactate or calcium gluconate by mouth. Twelve to 15 gm. per day in divided doses may be required. The oral calcium should be continued indefinitely or until the blood calcium and phosphorus levels return to normal. If the serum calcium does not respond to simple oral calcium therapy, parenteral injections of parathormone in doses of 100 units may be necessary to tide the patient over until vitamin D, administered in doses of from 50,000 to 300,000 units daily, becomes effective. This vitamin has little cumulative action, and once the proper dosage has been determined it does not tend to produce a dangerous hypercalcemia. Dihydrotachysterol (A.T. 10), a potent vitamin D derivative, has also been widely used for the treatment of chronic hypocalcemia

TABLE 11

Management of Parathyroid Tetany

1. Draw blood for serum calcium and phosphorus determinations.
2. Give 10 to 20 cc. of 10 per cent calcium gluconate intravenously.
3. Give calcium gluconate by mouth. Twelve or more grams in divided doses may be required daily.
4. Administer parathormone parenterally in doses of 100 units if symptoms are not relieved by calcium gluconate therapy.
5. Give vitamin D orally in doses of from 50,000 to 300,000 units daily. This will gradually abolish the need for parathormone.
6. If vitamin D does not prove adequate, dihydrotachysterol (A. T. 10) may be administered for maintenance therapy in oral doses of from 5 to 10 cc. initially, followed by 2 cc. twice weekly (see text for toxic effects).

N.B.: The majority of these patients recover promptly on calcium gluconate therapy alone, and the long acting agents should not be prescribed where calcium gluconate will suffice.

in oral doses of 5 to 10 cc. daily initially, followed by 2 cc. twice weekly. However, this drug has a definite cumulative action and its administration must be controlled by frequent serum calcium determinations. It is better to avoid its use where vitamin D therapy will suffice.

When the immediate emergency of tetany is over, it is helpful to ask the pathologist to examine the excised specimen again for parathyroid bodies. Unless several of these are found, the chances are excellent that the patient's serum calcium will quickly return to normal. Indeed, the majority of these patients recover promptly and completely on simple calcium gluconate therapy alone. For this reason one should not be stampeded into giving long-acting therapy in the acute emergency. If A.T. 10 is administered, one must wait much longer to learn whether or not the patient will have adequate parathyroid function.

RESPIRATORY OBSTRUCTION DURING OPERATION. In operations on the thyroid gland stridor may be present in some degree. This is, of course, disturbing to the operator. We have largely avoided this by the liberal use of the endotracheal tube.

POSTOPERATIVE RESPIRATORY OBSTRUCTION. This condition is, in the writer's opinion, the most dangerous complication associated with thyroidectomy. It is particularly likely to be disastrous because it often occurs when the patient is no longer under the alert observation of the operating team. It usually appears during the first 48 to 72 hours following operation and may be the result of edema in and around the larynx or, more likely, of hemorrhage. The onset is insidious. At first there may be no more than a subjective feeling of tightness in the neck and an objective appearance of fullness. Presently the patient becomes dyspneic and this may be the last warning before a terrifying state of

TABLE 12

STEPS IN TRACHEOTOMY

1. *Position:* Head over side of bed with neck hyperextended.
2. *Illumination:* The bed lamp may be satisfactory. If not, a goosenecked lamp may be available.
3. *Suction* is helpful.
4. *Tracheotomy equipment:* A complete tracheotomy set is desirable, but a scalpel or scissors, retractors, and a tracheotomy tube will suffice. In the absence of a tracheotomy tube, any tube which will keep the airway open should be used.
5. *Anesthesia:* In acute emergencies with severe anoxia no anesthesia is required. When time permits, local anesthesia is satisfactory.
6. *Skin incision:* If the circumstances permit niceties, we prefer a transverse incision for cosmetic reasons. If time is of the essence, a vertical incision over the trachea is the most efficient.
7. *Tracheal incision:* Aim for a point two or three rings below the cricoid cartilage. However, a precise site of entrance must always take second place to the necessity for establishing an opening in the trachea through which the patient can be oxygenated.
8. Secure tracheotomy tube in place by tying with hernia tape around neck.

respiratory distress and cyanosis suddenly intervenes. At the first appearance of any of these signs and symptoms hemorrhage should be suspected and the wound reopened if doubt exists. After several such experiences, an iron-clad rule has been made at the Hospital of the University of Pennsylvania that there must be a tracheotomy set-up present on each surgical ward at all times. Furthermore, the resident staff has been indoctrinated with the concept that the time to do a tracheotomy is when one is first forced to think of it. Only in this way can such patients be saved. It is admitted that an occasional patient will have an unnecessary tracheotomy performed, but in the long run this is a small price to pay for the lives which will be saved.

POSTOPERATIVE MYXEDEMA. The appearance of myxedema following therapy for thyrotoxicosis may prove to be more common after radioiodine than after subtotal thyroidectomy. In either case, the condition is managed with adequate doses of thyroid substance.

Carcinoma of the Thyroid

Carcinomas of the thyroid may be grouped broadly into papillary and nonpapillary types, but since it aids our concept of prognosis to group

THE THYROID GLAND

tumors according to their degree of malignancy, we have adopted the classification suggested by Shields Warren, which follows:

Tumors of low or potential malignancy
    Adenoma with blood vessel invasion
    Papillary cystadenoma with blood vessel invasion

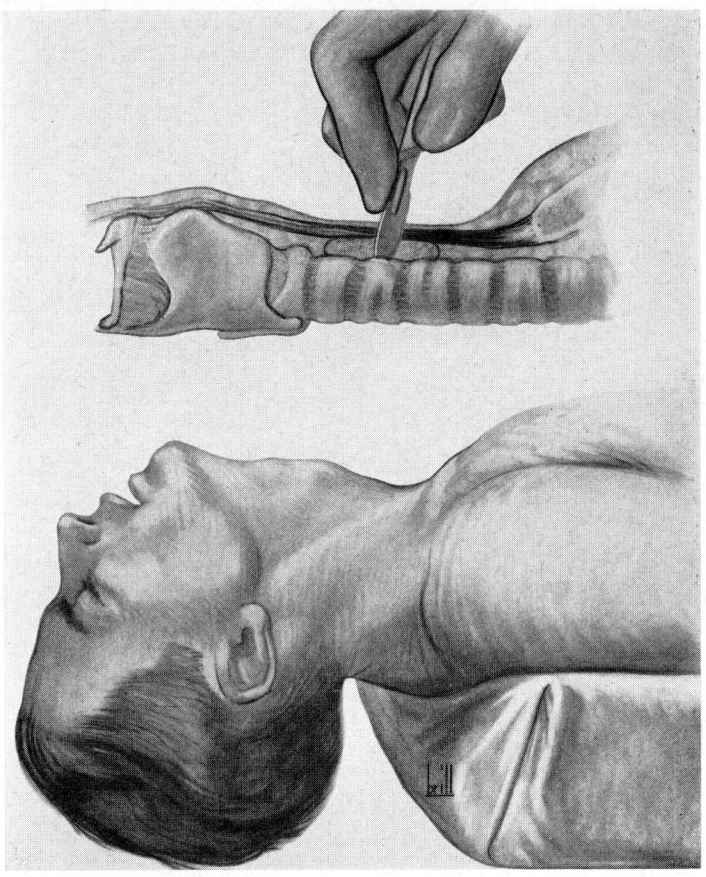

Fig. 28. Position and incision for tracheotomy. *Above:* Side view showing anterior incision in trachea. Only the tip of the knife should be inserted through tracheal ring. The thyroid isthmus is not often troublesome, unless the thyroid is enlarged, and it can usually be avoided. *Below:* Position showing neck hyperextended. This can be readily accomplished by holding the patient's head over the side of the bed.

Tumors of moderate malignancy
    Papillary adenocarcinoma
    Alveolar adenocarcinoma
    Hürthle cell adenocarcinoma
Tumors of high malignancy
    Small cell carcinoma (simple)
    Giant cell carcinoma

Epidermoid carcinoma
Fibrosarcoma
Lymphoma

One of the major difficulties confronting the thyroid pathologist is that of separating benign tumors from those of low or potential malignancy. This is obvious from the frequency of disagreement among reports from different clinics as to the incidence of this disease and, indeed, from differences in opinions concerning the same microscopic sections.

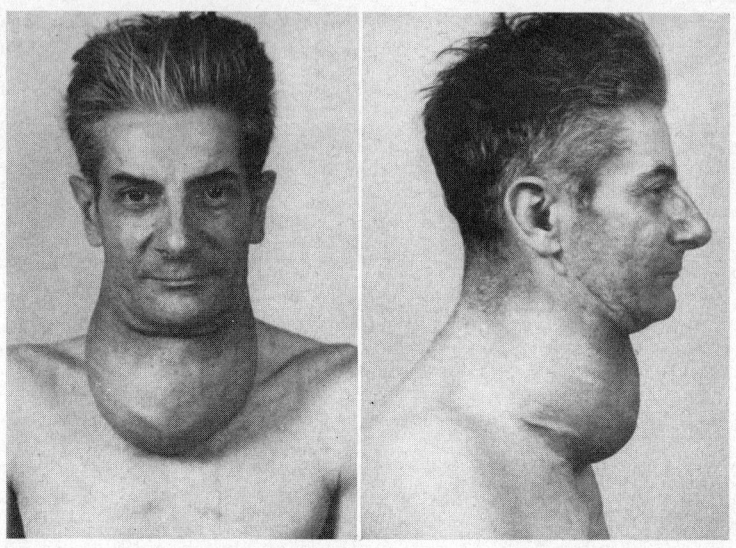

Fig. 29. Carcinoma of the thyroid in a goiter present for many years. This gland was hard, fixed, and was resected with considerable difficulty. The patient received roentgen therapy following operation.

Blood vessel invasion was first advanced as a criterion of malignancy by Graham in 1924, and Shields Warren has since examined it most carefully. In the latter's follow-up of 1080 cases in which he had found no blood vessel invasion, no case had developed evidence of malignancy in from two and one-half to seven years after operation. In the thirty-three cases in which blood vessel invasion had been found, two had died of cancer, one in ten months and another in two and one-half years. Later Lahey, Hare and Warren reported that less than 3 per cent of all adenomas have blood vessel invasion and that in only 10 per cent of those patients in whom blood vessel invasion has been found has definite clinical evidence of malignancy developed. Thus, the "benign adenomas" in which blood vessel invasion appears must be considered potentially malignant.

Papillary Adenocarcinoma. This is a very common type of thyroid cancer and, together with alveolar adenocarcinoma, it comprises ap-

THE THYROID GLAND 93

proximately two-thirds of all thyroid malignancy. The papillary adenocarcinoma is frequently found in the younger age groups, including individuals in their teens. It metastasizes most commonly to surrounding tissues and regional lymph nodes, more rarely to the skeleton and lungs. The microscopic picture is characterized by papillary projections exhibiting cytologic evidence of malignancy. These tumors are slow growing and have a rather good salvage rate if handled early and vigorously.

Alveolar Adenocarcinoma. This corresponds roughly to the malignant adenoma, or adenocarcinoma in fetal adenoma, and occurs more frequently in middle age. This tumor presents a variety of microscopic pictures, indicative of its origin from a fetal adenoma or from nodules of previously normal thyroid tissue. These lesions, too, metastasize to local lymph nodes, but they are also likely to metastasize to the skeleton, brain and viscera.

The other tumors listed in the classification of thyroid malignancies are much less commonly encountered. This is fortunate, since most of them are quite malignant and bear a very poor prognosis.

Treatment of Carcinoma of the Thyroid

While carcinoma of the thyroid is frequently slow growing and the immediate salvage rate is superior to that of many more malignant

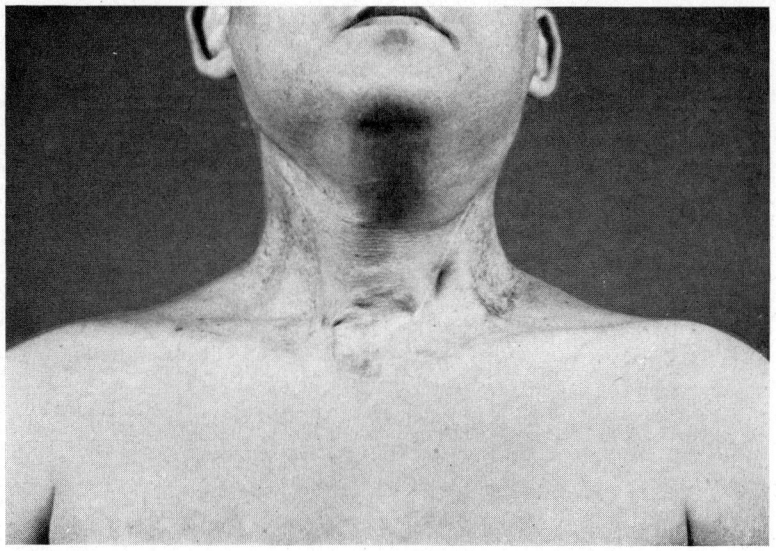

Fig. 30. Appearance of patient following bilateral radical neck dissection for carcinoma of the thyroid. (Courtesy of Dr. Henry P. Royster.)

tumors, patients with this disease are very likely to die of it eventually. Accordingly, every effort must be made to eradicate the disease totally when it is first discovered. If the presence of carcinoma is suspected at the time of operation, it can be made more certain by frozen section examination and a radical procedure can be carried out immediately. At the least this should include total lobectomy on the involved side combined with a radical neck dissection to remove adjacent strap muscles, the sternocleidomastoid muscle, the internal jugular vein, and all adjacent nodes and connective tissue en bloc. It is often necessary to sacrifice the recurrent nerve on the involved side. The initial operation affords the best opportunity for cure but, unfortunately, the presence of carcinoma may not be suspected until the paraffin sections of the tissue removed at the time of operation have been examined. In this case, if the entire lobe involved has not been removed the patient should be operated upon again and the procedure described above carried out. Lymph nodes containing metastases are not necessarily enlarged. We believe that following radical resection these patients should receive roentgen therapy.

Thyroid Carcinoma with Distant Metastases. If the patient has metastases in the lungs or skeleton at the time he is first seen, the only therapy likely to be of substantial benefit is that of radioactive iodine. The detailed technic of its use should be consulted in the appended references but, in brief, one gives a tracer dose of radioiodine by mouth twenty-four to forty-eight hours preceding operation at which a total thyroidectomy is done. The amount of radioactive iodine taken up by the malignant tissue from the thyroid is then determined by the radioautograph technic. If this uptake is adequate and if collateral evidence of functional activity of the metastases is obtained by placing a Geiger-Müller counter over these lesions, the patient may be given large doses of I^{131} with the hope that the metastases, wherever they may be, will take up this element and thus be destroyed by the internal irradiation. The rationale for doing a preliminary thyroidectomy is that this throws the entire TSH action on the metastases, resulting frequently in a greater I^{131} uptake by these lesions. There is also evidence that metastases can be stimulated to still further activity by the administration of thiouracil or/and TSH (Rawson). We have seen pulmonary metastases literally melt away in isolated instances.

Lateral Aberrant Thyroid. It is now generally conceded that in practically every instance thyroid carcinoma found in the neck lateral to the main thyroid gland is in reality a metastasis from a lesion situated in the lobe on the involved side. This condition is treated in the same manner as other thyroid carcinoma with metastasis.

Subacute Thyroiditis

This is a self-limited disease of uncertain etiology which runs a course of weeks or months and usually subsides without treatment (Crile). Associated with pain and tenderness, it responds readily to roentgen therapy and thyroidectomy is usually not indicated.

Struma Lymphomatosa (Hashimoto's Struma)

This may be a manifestation of systemic disease. It practically always occurs in women of middle age and the gross thyroid enlargement is strikingly characterized microscopically by extensive lymphoid infiltration. Treatment usually consists of liberal subtotal thyroidectomy, which relieves the pressure symptoms. Roentgen therapy is also effective.

Chronic Ligneous Thyroiditis (Riedel's Struma)

This is a condition which affects both sexes but is twice as common in women and usually occurs in middle age. The thyroid enlarges, becomes stony hard, and is firmly adherent to adjacent structures. The acinous elements of the gland are gradually replaced in large part by dense fibrotic tissue. The symptoms are chiefly those of pressure, dyspnea and dysphagia. The process is unilateral in about 50 per cent of cases. The problem in differential diagnosis is to rule out cancer; this is usually done at operation where as much of the mass as can be freed safely from the trachea, recurrent nerves and large vessels is resected. A second operation is rarely required and the development of hypothyroidism, which is hastened by operation, is treated with thyroid substance (Crile).

REFERENCES

Astwood, E. B.: Thiouracil treatment in hyperthyroidism. J. Clin. Endocrinol., *4:*229, 1944.
———: Treatment of hyperthyroidism with thiourea and thiouracil. J.A.M.A., *122:*78, 1943.
——— and Stanley, M. M.: Use of radioactive iodine in study of thyroid function in man. West. J. Surg., *55:*625, 1947.
———, Sullivan, J., Bissel, A., and Tyslowitz, R.: Action of certain sulfonamides and of thiourea upon function of the thyroid gland of the rat. Endocrinology, *32:*210, 1943.
Balls, K., Phillips, J., and Hardy, J. D.: Status of the conversion ratio as a measure of thyroid activity. Federation Proc., *10* (Part 1):9, 1951.
Benedict, F. G.: Degree of constancy in human basal metabolism. Am. J. Physiol., *110:*521, 1934.
Berlin, D. D., and Lahey, F. H.: Dissections of the recurrent and superior laryngeal nerves. Surg., Gynec. & Obst., *49:*102, 1929.
Boyd, W.: Surgical Pathology. 6th ed. Philadelphia, W. B. Saunders Company, 1947.
Cattell, R. B., and Morgan, E. S.: Recurrent hyperthyroidism; report of 306 cases operated upon from 1928–1937. Surg., Gynec. & Obst., *68:*347, 1939.
Chaikoff, I. L., Taurog, A., and Reinhardt, W. O.: The metabolic significance of protein-bound iodine of plasma: a study of its concentration under various conditions and its rate of formation as measured with radioactive iodine. Endocrinology, *40:*47, 1947.
Chapman, E. M., and Evans, R. D.: Treatment of hyperthyroidism with radioactive iodine. J.A.M.A. *131:*86, 1946.
——— and Evans, R. D.: Treatment of toxic goiters with radioactive iodine. M. Clin. North America, *33:*1211, 1949.
Clark, D. E., Moe, R. H., and Adams, E. E.: The rate of conversion of administered inorganic radioactive iodine into protein-bound iodine of plasma as an aid in the evaluation of thyroid function. Surgery, *26:*331, 1949.
Cole, W. H., Slaughter, D. F., and Rossiter, L. J.: Potential dangers of nontoxic nodular goiter. J.A.M.A., *127:*883, 1945.

Coller, F. A., and Maddock, W. G.: Water balance in patients with hyperthyroidism. West. J. Surg., *41*:438, 1933.
Cope, O., Rawson, R. W., and McArthur, J. W.: Hyperfunctioning single adenoma of thyroid. Surg., Gynec. & Obst., *84*:415, 1947.
Crile, G., and Crile, G., Jr.: A radical operation for malignant tumors of the thyroid gland. Surg., Gynec. & Obst., *64*:927, 1937.
Crile, G., Jr.: Practical Aspects of Thyroid Disease. Philadelphia, W. B. Saunders Company, 1949.
———: Papillary carcinoma of thyroid and lateral cervical region; so-called "Lateral aberrant thyroid." Surg., Gynec. & Obst., *85*:757, 1947.
———: Tumors of lateral aberrant thyroid origin. J.A.M.A., *113*:1094, 1939.
———, McCullagh, E. P., and Glasser, O.: Radioactive iodine in the treatment of hyperthyroidism. Cleveland Clin. Quart., *16*:1, 1949.
Curtis, G. M., and Fertman, M. B.: Blood iodine studies, an analysis of the blood iodine in thyroid disease. Arch. Surg., *50*:207, 1945.
Cutler, E. C., and Zollinger, R.: The surgical procedure for total thyroidectomy. Surg., Gynec. & Obst., *67*:69, 1938.
DeCourcy, J. L., and DeCourcy, C. B.: Pathology and Surgery of Thyroid Disease. Springfield, Illinois, Charles C Thomas, 1949.
Dinsmore, R. S., and Crile, G., Jr.: Thyroid problems and end-results of operations on the thyroid gland. S. Clin. North America, *15*:859, 1935.
Dobyns, B. M.: Thyroid nodules, benign and malignant; observations on their function. M. Clin. North America, *33*:1225, 1949.
Franklin, A. L., Lerner, S. R., and Chaikoff, I. L.: The effect of thiouracil on the formation of thyroxine and diiodotyrosine by thyroid gland of the rat with radioactive iodine as an indicator. Endocrinology, *34*:265, 1944.
Frazier, C. H., and Brown, R. B.: The thyroid and the liver. West. J. Surg., *43*:636, 1935.
Friedberg, C. K., and Sohval, A. R.: Occurrence and pathogenesis of cardiac hypertrophy in Graves' disease. Am. Heart J., *13*:599, 1937.
Goetsch, E.: Recurrent nerve injury. Ann. Surg., *108*:559, 1938.
———: A new concept regarding the origin of so-called primary carcinoma of the hyperplastic thyroid. Ibid., *118*:843, 1943.
Graham, A.: Criteria of malignancy. Radiology, *37*:521, 1941.
———: Malignant epithelial tumors of the thyroid. Surg., Gynec. & Obst., *39*:781, 1924.
———: Malignant tumors of thyroid; epithelial types. Ann. Surg., *82*:30, 1925.
———: Riedel's struma in contrast to struma lymphomatosa (Hashimoto). West J. Surg., *39*:681, 1931.
———: Struma lymphomatosa (Hashimoto). Tr. Am. A. Study Goiter, 1940, p. 222.
——— and McCullagh, E. P.: Atrophy and fibrosis associated with lymphoid tissue in the thyroid, Struma lymphomatosa (Hashimoto). Arch. Surg., *22*:548, 1931.
Hamilton, J. G., and Soley, M. H.: Studies in iodine metabolism by the use of a new radioactive isotope of iodine. Am. J. Physiol., *127*:557, 1939.
——— and Soley, M. H.: Studies in iodine metabolism of thyroid gland in situ by use of radioiodine in normal subjects and in patients with various types of goiter. Am. J. Physiol., *131*:135, 1940.
Hardy, J. D., and Riegel, C.: The laboratory diagnosis of hyperthyroidism. A practical analysis of current methods with a presentation of illustrative cases. Am. J. M. Sc., *221*:359, 1951.
———, Riegel, C., and Erisman, E. P.: Experience with protein-bound iodine (PBI); effect of ACTH and cortisone on thyroid function. Ibid., 219:581, 1950.
Hare, H. F.: Radiation treatment of carcinoma of the thyroid. Am. J. Roentgenol., *46*:451, 1947.
Heinbecker, P.: The pathogenesis of hyperthyroidism. Ann. Surg., *130*:804, 1949.
Hertz, S., and Roberts, A.: Radioactive iodine as indicator in thyroid physiology; iodine collection as criterion of thyroid function in rabbits injected with thyrotropic hormone. Endocrinology, *29*:82, 1941.
——— and Roberts, A.: Radioactive iodine in the study of thyroid physiology. VII. The use of radioactive iodine therapy in hyperthyroidism. J.A.M.A., *131*:81, 1946.

Hertz, S., Roberts, A., and Salter, W. T.: Radioactive iodine as an indicator in thyroid physiology. IV. The metabolism of iodine in Graves' disease. J. Clin. Investigation, 21:25, 1942.

Hertzler, A. E.: Surgical Pathology of the Thyroid Gland. Philadelphia, J. B. Lippincott Co., 1936.

Hinton, J. W., and Lord, J. W., Jr.: Is surgery indicated in all cases of nodular goiter, toxic and nontoxic? J.A.M.A., 129:605, 1945.

Horn, R. C.: Personal communication.

Hurxthal, L. M.: Blood cholesterol in thyroid disease; myxedema and hypercholesteremia. Arch. Int. Med., 53:762, 1934.

Johnson, J., and Kirby, C. K.: The surgical treatment of ventricular fibrillation. Ann. Surg., 134:672, 1951.

Keating, F. R., Jr., Power, M. H., Berkson, J., and Haines, S. F.: The urinary excretion of radioiodine in various thyroid states. J. Clin. Investigation, 26:1138, 1947.

King, B. T., and Rosellini, L. J.: Treatment of acute thyroiditis with thiouracil; preliminary report. J.A.M.A., 129:267, 1945.

King, W. L. M., and Pemberton, J. deJ.: So-called lateral aberrant thyroid tumors. Surg., Gynec. & Obst., 74:991, 1942.

Kunde, M. M.: Studies on metabolism; experimental hyperthyroidism. Am. J. Physiol., 82:195, 1927.

Lahey, F. H.: A method of removing discrete adenomata of the thyroid. Ann. Surg., 86:31, 1927.

———: Carcinoma of thyroid. Am. J. Roentgenol., 46:469, 1941.

———: Combination of Lugol's solution with thiouracil in preoperative preparations of patients with toxic goiter. Lahey Clin. Bull., 4:2, 1944.

———: Goiter incisions. Ann. Surg., 117:332, 1943.

———: Intrathoracic goiter. J.A.M.A., 113:1098, 1939.

———: Routine dissection and demonstration of recurrent laryngeal nerve in subtotal thyroidectomy. Surg., Gynec. & Obst., 66:775, 1938.

———: The reduction of mortality in hyperthyroidism. New England J. Med., 213:475, 1935.

——— and Ficarra, B. J.: Lateral aberrant thyroid. Surg., Gynec. & Obst., 82:705, 1946.

——— and Hare, H. F.: Malignant adenomas of the thyroid. J.A.M.A., 145:689, 1951.

———, Hare, H. F., and Warren, S.: Carcinoma of thyroid. Ann. Surg., 112:977, 1940.

Leiter, L., Seidlin, S. M., Marinelli, L. D., and Baumann, E. J.: Adenocarcinoma of thyroid with hyperthyroidism and functional metastases; studies with thiouracil and radioiodine. J. Clin. Endocrinol., 6:247, 1946.

McArthur, J. W., Rawson, R. W., Fluharty, R. G., and Means, J. H.: The urinary excretion of radioactive iodine as an aid in the diagnosis of hyperthyroidism. Ann. Int. Med. 29:229, 1948.

McClintock, J. C., and Wright, A. W.: Riedel's struma and struma lymphomatosa (Hashimoto); comparative study. Ann. Surg., 106:11, 1937.

Man, E. B., and Peters, J. P.: Artifactual values of serum precipitable iodine. J. Lab. & Clin. Med., 35:280, 1950.

Marine, D.: Etiology and prevention of simple goiter. Medicine, 3:453, 1924.

Means, J. H.: The Thyroid and Its Diseases. Philadelphia, J. B. Lippincott Co., 1948.

——— and Aub, J. C.: Basal metabolism in hypothyroidism. Arch. Int. Med., 24:404, 1919.

——— and Lerman, J.: Action of iodine in thyrotoxicosis with special reference to refractoriness: J.A.M.A., 104:969, 1935.

Morton, M. E., Chaikoff, I. L., Reinhardt, W. O., and Anderson, E.: Radioactive iodine as indicator of metabolism of iodine, formation of thyroxine and diiodotyrosine by completely thyroidectomized animal. J. Biol. Chem., 147:757, 1943.

———, Perlman, I., and Chaikoff, I. L.: Radioactive iodine as an indicator of the metabolism of iodine. III The effect of thyrotropic hormone on the turnover of thyroxine and diiodotyrosine in the thyroid gland and plasma. Ibid., 140:603, 1941.

Pemberton, J. deJ.: Recurring exophthalmic goiter; its relation to amount of tissue preserved in operation on thyroid gland. J.A.M.A., 94:1483, 1930.

Perkin, H. J.: Value of blood iodine estimations in treatment of clinical hyperthyroidism. S. Clin. North America, 16:1509, 1936.
Peters, J. P., and Man, E. B.: The significance of serum cholesterol in thyroid disease. J. Clin. Investigation, 29:1, 1950.
Plummer, H. S.: Results of administration of iodine to patients having exophthalmic goiter. J.A.M.A., 80:1955, 1923.
Rawson, R. W.: Malignancy of the thyroid; in Means, J. H.: The Thyroid and Its Diseases. Philadelphia, J. B. Lippincott Co., 1948, p. 460.
———: Pathology of the thyroid; in Means, J. H.: The Thyroid and Its Diseases. Philadelphia, J. B. Lippincott Co., 1948,
———, Evans, R. D., Means, J. H., Peacock, W. C., Lerman, J., and Cortell, R. E.: Action of thiouracil upon thyroid gland in Graves' disease. J. Clin. Endocrinol., 4:1, 1944.
Rogers, W. F., Asper, S. P., Jr., and Williams, R. H.: Clinical significance of malignant neoplasma of the thyroid gland. New England J. Med., 237:569, 1947.
Rundle, F. F.: Development and course of exophthalmus and ophthalmoplegia in Graves' disease with special reference to effect of thyroidectomy. Clin. Sci., 5:177, 1945.
Salter, W. T., Bassett, A. M., and Sappington, T. S.: Protein-bound iodine in blood; its relation to thyroid function in 100 clinical cases. Am. J. M. Sc., 202:527, 1941.
Schilling, J. A.: Struma lymphomatosa, struma fibrosa and thyroiditis. Surg., Gynec. & Obst., 81:533, 1945.
Seidlin, S. M., Marinelli, L. D., and Oshry, E.: Radioactive iodine therapy; effect on functioning metastases of adenocarcinoma of the thyroid. J.A.M.A., 132:838, 1946.
Sheline, G. E., and Clark, D. E.: Index of thyroid function: estimation by rate of organic binding of I^{131}. J. Lab. & Clin. Med., 36:450, 1950.
———, Moore, M. C., Kappas, A., and Clark, D. E.: A correlation between the serum protein-bound iodine and the radioiodine conversion ratio in various thyroid states. J. Clin. Endocrinol., 11:91, 1951.
Smith, P. E., and Smith, I. P.: Repair and activation of thyroid in hypophysectomized tadpole by parenteral administration of fresh anterior lobe bovine hypophysis. J. M. Research, 43:267, 1922.
Stanbury, J. B.: Problems in the diagnosis of thyrotoxicosis. M. Clin. North America, 33:1231, 1949.
Taurog, A., and Chaikoff, I. L.: Nature of plasma iodine. J. Biol. Chem., 171:439, 1947.
Thompson, W. O., Morris, A. E., and Thompson, P. K.: Thyrotoxicosis following subtotal thyroidectomy for exophthalmic goiter. Arch. Int. Med., 46:946, 1930.
Warren, S.: Classification of tumors of the thyroid. Am. J. Roentgenol., 46:447, 1941.
———: Significance of invasion of blood vessels in adenomas of the thyroid gland. Arch. Path., 11:255, 1931.
Werner, S. C., Quimby, E. H., and Schmidt, C.: Clinical experiences in diagnosis and treatment of thyroid disorders with radioactive iodine (eight day half-life). Radiology, 51:564, 1948.
Winkler, A. W., Riggs, D. S., Thompson, K. W., and Man, E. B.: Serum iodine in hyperthyroidism with particular reference to effects of subtotal thyroidectomy. J. Clin. Investigation, 25:404, 1946.

CHAPTER 8

HYPERPARATHYROIDISM

Although von Recklinghausen first described the tumors, cysts, and generalized decalcification of osteitis fibrosa cystica generalisata in 1891, it was not until 1925 that Mandl, a Vienna surgeon, proved the parathyroid etiology of this disease by excising an adenoma and demonstrating the recalcification of the demineralized bones. At almost the same time DuBois, aware that the clinical picture in his patient was similar to that produced by the administration of parathormone, arrived at the correct diagnosis of a parathyroid adenoma on the basis of this physiologic reasoning. In the years that followed Albright and his associates made exhaustive studies of the physiology of the parathyroid glands, and to these men and to Collip we are indebted for a very considerable part of our knowledge of parathyroid disease.

Functioning adenomas of the parathyroids are not rare. Cases are being reported in increasing numbers throughout the United States, and it is evident that the frequency with which accurate diagnoses of excessive parathyroid activity are made will be directly proportional to the care with which the condition is sought. In 1949 Rienhoff was able to obtain reports of 597 proved cases. Of these, the group at the Massachusetts General Hospital had treated 104 cases and the group at the Mayo Clinic, 106. Although bone demineralization has been the pathology most frequently associated with this disease in physicians' minds, it is a less sensitive indicator of hyperparathyroidism than is the presence of renal stones. Albright believes that about 10 per cent of all renal stones have excessive parathyroid activity as an underlying etiology.

PHYSIOLOGY OF THE PARATHYROIDS

Normal Regulation of Parathyroid Activity. The parathyroid glands exert their endocrinologic action through the elaboration of parathormone, which was first isolated by Collip in 1925. The regulation of the rate of formation of this hormone has been the subject of many interesting studies. Carnes, Pappenheimer and Stoerk demonstrated that rats fed a diet low in calcium developed marked enlargement of the parathyroid glands and that a diet high in calcium but low in phosphorus resulted in a significant reduction in parathyroid volume in comparison with stock diet controls. The addition of gradual increments of potassium phosphate to the low phosphorus, high calcium diet increased the serum phosphate proportionately and caused a corresponding increase in parathyroid volume. These workers also found that large doses of viosterol further reduced the size of the parathyroids on a low phosphorus diet, at the same time raising the serum levels of both calcium and phosphorus. Viosterol inhibited the hyperplasia produced by a low calcium diet. Patt, Wallerstein and Luckhardt also showed that parathyroid hypertrophy could be produced by a low calcium diet. These authors demonstrated that the perfusion of the isolated thyro-parathyroid apparatus of the dog with decalcified blood resulted in a perfusate which would cause a rise in the serum calcium when injected into normal dogs. This did not result when the perfusion was done with normal blood. While no simple formula has yet been devised quantitatively to relate parathyroid

TABLE 13

ACTION OF PARATHORMONE

(After Aub, Cope)

---

1. The hormone acts on the renal tubules to increase the excretion of phosphorus.
2. In an attempt to preserve the serum phosphorus level this ion is mobilized from the bones, resulting in a demineralization of these structures.
3. The excessive mobilization of calcium phosphate results in an elevated serum calcium level.

---

volume to serum calcium under all conditions, the level of serum calcium is surely important in regulating the rate of parathormone formation. The liberation of the parathyroid hormone appears to be independent of nervous control, and the control of the parathyroids by the pituitary has not been established.

Mode of Action of Parathormone. There has been much discussion as to the site of action of parathormone. Recent studies with P^{32} (Tweedy, Chilcote and Patras) have supported the earlier view of Aub and associates that the parathyroid glands have their primary influence on phosphorus metabolism through a direct action on the kidney tubules to increase the excretion of phosphorus. These workers found that following thyroparathyroidectomy the early diminution in urinary and fecal excretion of administered phosphate tagged with P^{32} could be reversed within one hour by the injection of parathyroid extract. After bilateral nephrectomy this material had no effect on the distribution, retention, or excretion of P^{32}. These findings are strong support for a direct renal effect of parathormone, but they cannot in themselves disprove the view that the parathyroids may also influence osteoclastic activity in the bones.

PATHOLOGIC LESIONS IN HYPERPARATHYROIDISM

Primary Hyperparathyroidism. The lesions found in states of primary hyperparathyroidism are to be found in the parathyroid, the skeleton

HYPERPARATHYROIDISM

and the kidneys. The site of the excessive parathormone formation is almost invariably a functioning parathyroid tumor which may lie either in the neck or in the mediastinum. More than one tumor may be present, but usually only one parathyroid is enlarged. The excessive hormonal activity results in demineralization of the skeleton with cyst formation, pathologic fractures and other changes associated with osteitis fibrosa cystica (von Recklinghausen's disease). In approximately 30 per cent of cases of primary hyperparathyroidism the excessive hypercalcinuria results in the formation of renal stones, and the renal damage secondary to nephrolithiasis very often leads to uremia if the process is not reversed early.

In addition to functioning tumors, the parathyroid glands may at times exhibit benign nonfunctioning tumors, cysts or malignant changes.

Secondary Hyperparathyroidism. This condition is the result of a diffuse cellular hyperplasia of the parathyroid glands secondary to impaired renal function. The currently accepted theory is that in patients with chronic renal failure phosphate is not excreted in normal amounts and its concentration in body fluids rises. The rise in the phosphate ion concentration depresses the calcium ion to below normal levels and this in turn calls forth a compensatory overactivity of the parathyroid glands in an attempt to maintain the normal calcium level (Cope). This cellular hyperplasia is not uncommon in chronic renal insufficiency and this has been well documented by Pappenheimer and Wilens and by Castleman and Mallory. An associated demineralization of bones in childhood is sometimes referred to as "renal rickets."

In the presence of extensive renal damage it may be difficult, if not impossible, to distinguish between primary and secondary hyperparathyroidism. Cope points out that in the latter instance the serum calcium should theoretically never go above normal, for as soon as the normal level is reached the compensatory mechanism should cease. However, with progressive impairment of renal function in primary hyperparathyroidism the increasing phosphate retention might depress the serum calcium to normal or even below. Under such circumstances surgical resection of a parathyroid tumor or parathyroid hyperplasia would be contraindicated.

THE DIAGNOSIS OF PRIMARY HYPERPARATHYROIDISM

The presence of a functioning parathyroid tumor may be suspected from symptoms resulting from the chemical changes in the blood and urine, among which may be muscular atony, weakness, fatigue, constipation, anorexia, weight loss, nausea, polyuria and polydipsia. Keating found polyuria and polydipsia conspicuous in 46 per cent of his cases, and at times these symptoms may be so severe as to suggest the diagnosis of diabetes insipidus. Nevertheless, these symptoms have rarely been sufficient to result in a diagnosis of hyperparathyroidism prior to the development of renal or skeletal complications. The renal complications are the result of a deposition of calcium in the kidneys and may result in pain, infection or uremia. The demineralization of the bones may result in symptoms varying from vague, insignificant aches to real disability and pain accompanying the pathologic fractures, cysts, tumors and deformities which occur in the classic bone disease.

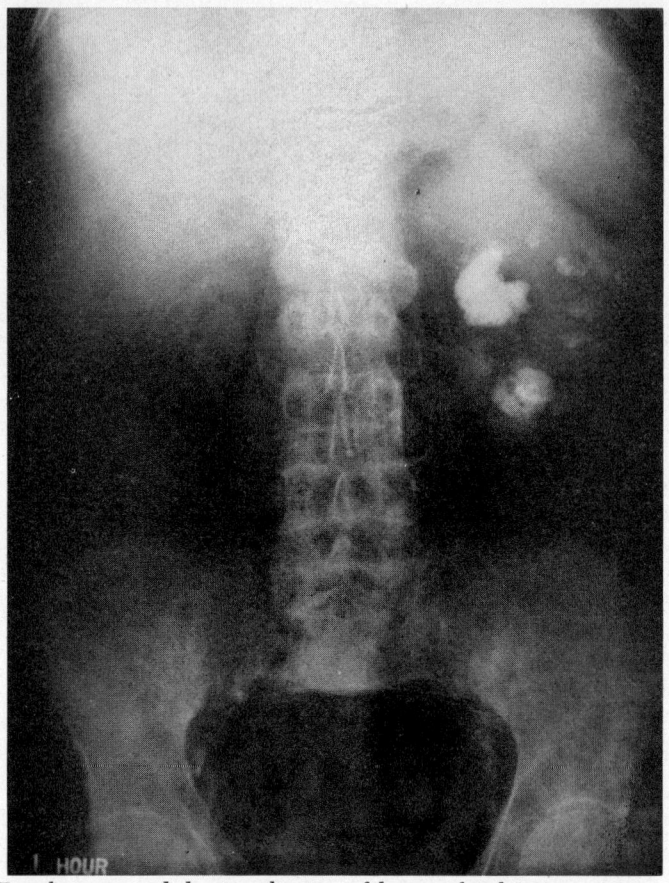

Fig. 31. Renal stones and demineralization of bones of pelvis in patient with hyperparathyroidism.

Serum Calcium Level. The ultimate diagnosis rests upon the laboratory demonstration of hypercalcemia, hypophosphatemia and hypercalcinuria. The normal serum calcium level is 10 ±1 mg. per 100 cc. For the diagnosis of hyperparathyroidism this value will usually be greater than 12.0 or 12.5 mg. Nevertheless, this level is not always reached even in the presence of hyperparathyroidism and, if present, it may not be present constantly. In twelve of twenty-four cases Keating found that the average concentration of serum calcium was less than 12.5 mg. per 100 cc.; in four cases the average level fell within the normal range; and in seven cases one or more determinations fell within the normal range. *Repeated calcium determinations over a period of weeks or months may be necessary to detect the hypercalcemia of hyperparathyroidism.*

The total concentration of serum calcium is dependent on the serum protein concentration and for this reason both values must be deter-

TABLE 14

Findings in Hyperparathyroidism

BONES	KIDNEYS
1. Pathologic fractures 2. Cyst formation	1. Stone formation (10 per cent of renal stones are associated with parathyroid adenomas) 2. Chronic infection secondary to stones 3. Late: renal failure (frequent cause of death)
BLOOD	URINE
1. Serum calcium level elevated (normal 10±1 mg. per 100 cc.) 2. Serum phosphorus level decreased normal 3.5±0.5 mg. per 100 cc.) 3. Alkaline phosphatase increased	1. Excessive calcium excretion (greater than 200 mg. per 24 hours on a low calcium diet)

mined. Calcium proteinate varies with alterations in serum protein and is not primarily affected by the parathyroid hormone, whereas ionic calcium is specifically affected. Thus, patients with a lowered serum protein level and a normal total serum calcium level may still have an increased ionic calcium level caused by excessive parathyroid activity. While these calcium fractions cannot be readily determined, their rela-

TABLE 15

Differential Diagnosis of Bone Lesions in Hyperparathyroidism

(After Jaffe)

1. Adolescent rickets, osteomalacia, or idiopathic steatorrhea
2. Senile osteoporosis
3. Carcinosis of the skeleton
4. Multiple myeloma
5. Paget's disease
6. Fibrous dysplasia of bone

tive concentrations can be estimated by the use of a nomogram prepared by McLean and Hastings. For example, the hypercalcemia of multiple myeloma or of sarcoidosis would be found to be paralleled by a rise in serum protein, indicating that the increased calcium level was due to the increased serum protein. A lowered serum protein level could theoretically mask the hypercalcemia of hyperparathyroidism, but in actual practice this is rarely encountered.

Inorganic Phosphorus Level of Serum. The serum level of inorganic phosphorus is normally 3.5 ±0.5mg. per 100 cc. The level is decreased in hyperparathyroidism. Although the average diminution is small, Cope has stated that in mild cases where the blood calcium level is borderline the phosphorus level may be of more help than the calcium level. A persistently low fasting phosphorus level, even in the presence of a normal blood calcium level, is held to be diagnostic provided there is an increased urinary excretion of calcium.

Urinary Calcium Excretion. Patients with hyperparathyroidism excrete excessive amounts of calcium in the urine. On a low calcium diet, of which that described by Bauer and Aub is satisfactory, the normal calcium excretion is less than 100 mg. per twenty-four hours and values greater than 200 mg. are abnormal. A measurement less exacting than the balance study and more easily employed clinically is the gross test (Barney and Sulkowitch) which consists of adding a buffer oxalate mixture to an aliquot of a twenty-four hour urine collection. If the patient has been on a low calcium diet (no milk or milk products) for three days, more than a trace of calcium precipitate suggests hyperparathyroidism and, if such calciuria persists, either hyperparathyroidism or some other cause for it exists (Cope).

Serum Alkaline Phosphatase. The serum alkaline phosphatase is usually elevated in hyperparathyroidism, but this is likely due to the bone disease and not to the hyperparathyroidism per se, since long after the serum calcium and phosphorus levels and the urinary calcium excretion have returned to normal the serum phosphatase may remain elevated.

MANAGEMENT OF PRIMARY HYPERPARATHYROIDISM

The treatment of primary hyperparathyroidism is surgical excision of the adenoma. A medical regimen consisting of a diet high in calcium will recalcify bones, but at the same time it increases the likelihood of renal stones. Roentgen therapy has proved unsatisfactory.

Operative Considerations

Location of Tumors. In 1931 Walton reported operations upon four patients with hyperparathyroidism due to adenomas of the parathyroid glands, and was the first to call attention to the importance of searching for abnormal parathyroid tissue in regions other than about the thyroid gland. In two of his patients parathyroid glands had been mechanically displaced from their original positions, and he noted that in such displacements the original vascular pedicle connecting the tumor to the thyroid artery was preserved. In 1934 and 1936, Churchill and Cope for the first time correlated the various locations in which adenomas were found with the embryogenesis of the parathyroid glands. Churchill further postulated that the parathyroid glands would probably be found within the limits of the tubular fascial structure of the neck bounded

HYPERPARATHYROIDISM

anteriorly by the deep layer of the middle cervical fascia and posteriorly by the prevertebral fascia. Surgeons were led to perform a systematic surgical dissection of the cervical region as well as of the posterior

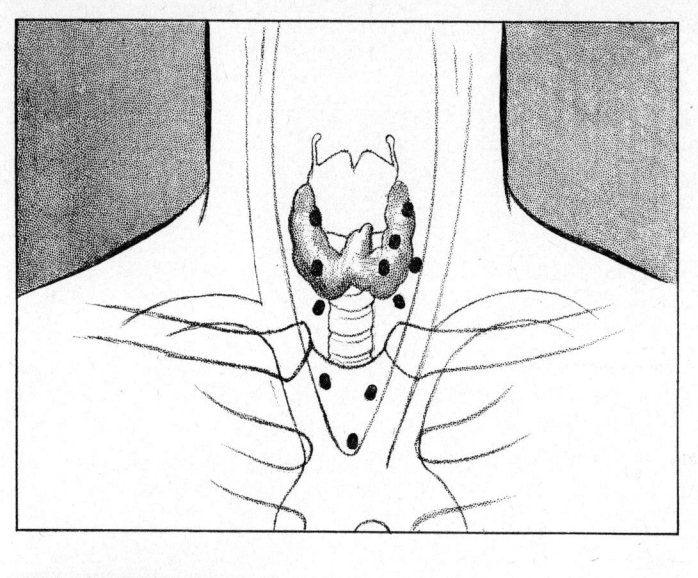

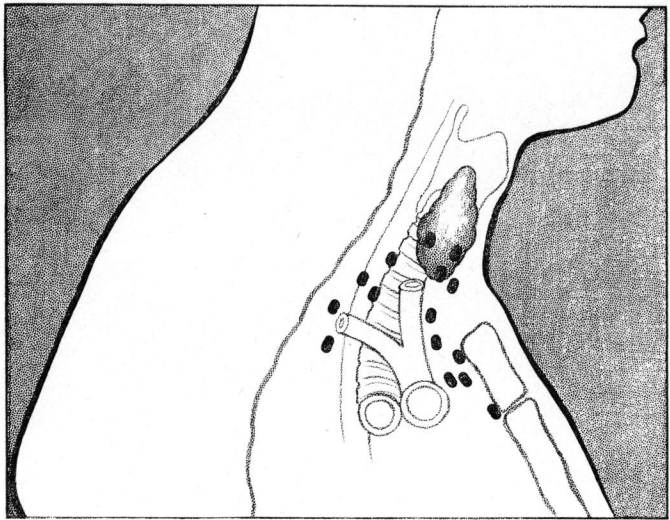

Fig. 32. Locations of parathyroid tumors in the neck and mediastinum. (Modified from Rienhoff, W. F.: Ann. Surg., *131*:917, 1950; J. B. Lippincott Company.)

superior and anterior superior mediastinum. This placed the search for parathyroid tumors on an embryologic as well as an anatomic basis.

Surgical Technic. An adequate search for a parathyroid adenoma presupposes a knowledge of the appearance of the normal parathyroids. Cope has emphasized the importance of careful study at the operating

106   SURGERY AND THE ENDOCRINE SYSTEM

table, in the postmortem room, and in the anatomic laboratory. First the neck is explored through a collar incision and with a bloodless field. After reflection of the skin flaps and platysma and division of the strap muscles, a meticulous and systematic course should be followed. Care is exercised to avoid cutting into the thyroid gland with resultant bleeding.

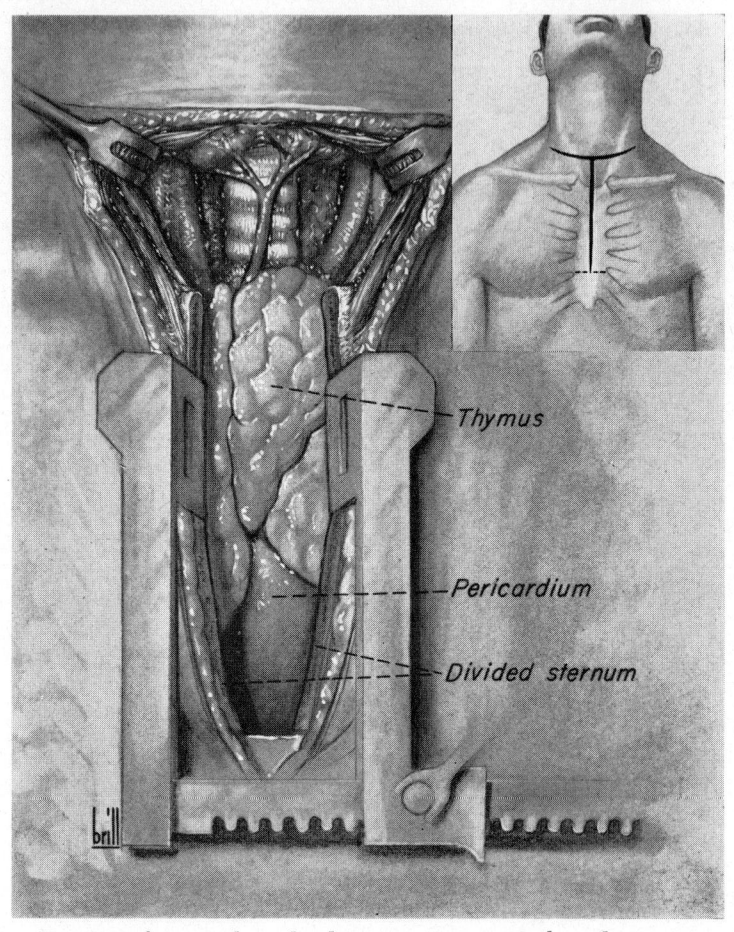

Fig. 33. Exposure for parathyroid adenomas. *Insert:* Neck and sternum incision. *Below:* Exposure of thymus and anterior mediastinum by division of sternum.

Retraction of this structure may be accompanied with traction sutures. The upper parathyroids are far more constant in position than are the lower ones, and it is advisable to search for these glands first. When they are found and are normal, they should not be removed. Atrophy of the located parathyroids suggests the presence elsewhere of a hyperfunctioning adenoma. If the superior parathyroids present no abnormality, the search for the inferior parathyroids is begun in the same meticulous manner. If these are not found in the neck they are searched for in the

HYPERPARATHYROIDISM

posterior superior mediastinum. If one or both still cannot be found, the sternum is split and the superior anterior mediastinum is examined. This may be done at a second operation if surgical judgment so dictates. The adenoma may be intimately associated with the thymus gland and, indeed, may lie within the thymus substance.

The exposure of the normal parathyroid glands is important in excluding those specific sites as locations for the adenoma. Furthermore, there may be present more than one adenoma. There may be more

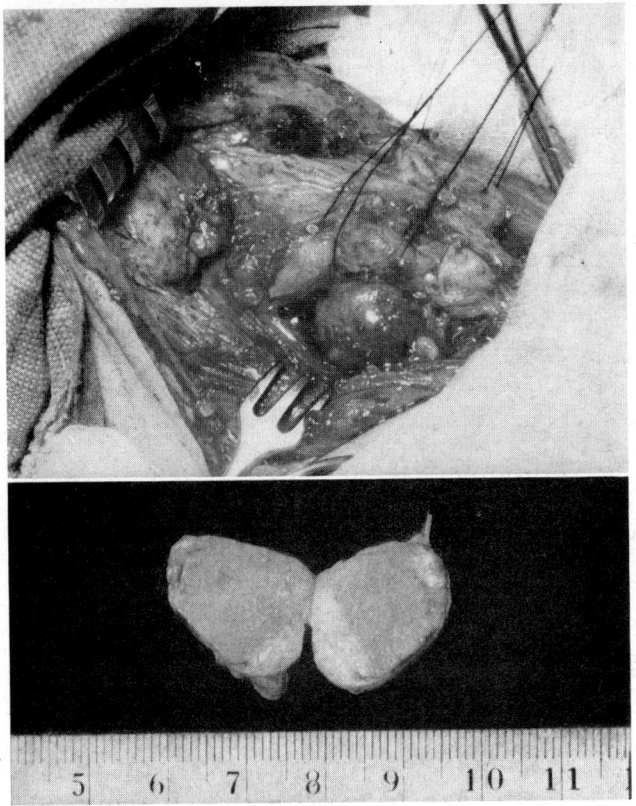

Fig. 34. Parathyroid adenoma in situ and after excision. (Courtesy of Dr. Henry P. Royster.)

than four parathyroid glands, but this is rare. Rienhoff warns against excision of the thymus if no adenoma is found there. It may contain normal parathyroid tissue. He also advises investigation of thyroid nodules. In two of his twenty-seven cases the parathyroid adenoma was intrathyroid. Approximately 80 per cent of adenomas are found in the cervical region and in the posterior superior mediastinum, but the adenomas located in the anterior mediastinum are the ones which are most frequently missed. Of nine cases referred to the Massachusetts General Hospital after an unsuccessful search elsewhere, six had tumors in the anterior mediastinum, one had a tumor in the posterior mediastinum and two had tumors in the neck (Cope).

In 1947 Black and Sprague reported the first case of hyperparathyroidism due to a diffuse primary hypertrophy and hyperplasia of the parathyroid glands recognized and treated surgically at the Mayo Clinic. The right superior and inferior and the left inferior parathyroid glands were resected. The left superior parathyroid gland, whose weight was estimated at about 300 mg., was preserved and the patient was apparently cured. In general, however, it is wise to be extremely conservative in reaching a diagnosis of primary hyperplasia, lest normal parathyroid glands be removed and an adenoma be overlooked. If primary hyperplasia is encountered, partial resection of the large parathyroid glands should be performed, leaving between 30 and 200 mg. of hyperplastic tissue (Albright). Care should be taken to preserve the blood supply of the tissue left behind.

Postoperative Care. The problem most likely to arise following the removal of a functioning adenoma is hypocalcemic tetany. This possibility must be anticipated and, if necessary, the patient should be treated with oral and intravenous calcium, parathormone and vitamin D (as outlined under complications of thyroidectomy in the previous chapter). The normal parathyroid glands often will have atrophied in the presence of the excessive parathormone secretion of the tumor and will require time to regain their normal function. In the interim the patient can be supported with substitution therapy.

Prognosis Following Removal of the Adenoma. The prognosis is largely dependent upon whether all the adenomata are removed and upon the state of the renal function at the time the patient is operated upon. In Rienhoff's series almost all the patients had irreversible and irremedial renal complications at the time of operation; these persisted following an operation in which the hyperparathyroidism was corrected. At the time he published his report, ten of his twenty-six cases had died and this 34.7 per cent mortality was expected to increase. Royster, in an experience with nineteen cases, reported only one death, but a number of his patients had badly damaged kidneys. It is imperative to make the diagnosis of hyperparathyroidism early. Only in this way can the patients be operated upon and the condition corrected before severe renal damage has occurred.

REFERENCES

Albright, F.: The parathyroids—physiology and therapeutics. J.A.M.A., *117*:527, 1941.
——, Bauer, W., Ropes, M., and Aub., J. C.: Studies of carcinoma and protein metabolism. IV. The effect of the parathyroid hormone. J. Clin. Investigation, 7:139, 1929.
——, Baird, P. C., Cope, O., and Bloomberg, E.: Studies on the physiology of the parathyroid glands. IV. Renal complications of hyperparathyroidism. Am. J. M. Sc., *187*:49, 1934.

Albright, F., Sulkowitch, H. W., and Bloomberg, E.: Hyperparathyroidism due to idiopathic hypertrophy (hyperplasia) of parathyroid tissue. Arch. Int. Med., 62:199, 1938.
———: Some medical aspects of the renal stone problem. New England J. Med., 217:1063, 1937.
———, Baird, P. C., Cope, O., and Bloomberg, E.: Studies on the physiology of the parathyroid glands; renal complications of hyperparathyroidism. Am. J. M. Sc., 187:49, 1934.
Alexander, H. B., Pemberton, J. deJ., Kepler, E. J., and Broders, A. C.: Functional parathyroid tumors and hyperparathyroidism; clinical and pathologic considerations. Am. J. Surg., 65:157, 1944.
Aub, J. C.: Calcium and phosphorus metabolism. Harvey Lect., 1928–1929, p. 151, 1930.
———, Bauer, W., Heath, C., and Ropes, M.: Studies of carcinoma and protein metabolism. III. The effects of the thyroid hormone and thyroid disease. J. Clin. Investigation, 7:97, 1929.
Barney, J. D., and Sulkowitch, H. W.: Progress in the management of urinary calculi. J. Urology, 37:746, 1937.
Barr, D. P., Bulger, H. A., and Dixon, H. H.: Hyperparathyroidism. J.A.M.A., 92:951, 1929.
Bauer, W., Albright, F., and Aub, J.: Studies of calcium and phosphorus metabolism. I. The calcium excretion of normal individuals on a low calcium diet, also data on a case of pregnancy. J. Clin. Investigation, 7:75, 1929.
——— and Aub, J. C.: Studies of inorganic salt metabolism. I. The ward routine and methods. J. Am. Dietet. A., 3:106, 1927.
Black, B. M., and Sprague, R. G.: Hyperparathyroidism due to diffuse primary hypertrophy and hyperplasia of the parathyroid glands: report of case. Proc. Staff Meet., Mayo Clin., 22:73, 1947.
Carnes, W. H., Pappenheimer, A. M., and Stoerk, H. C.: Value of parathyroid glands in relation to dietary calcium and phosphorus. Proc. Soc. Exper. Biol. & Med., 51:314, 1942.
Castleman, B., and Mallory, T. B.: The pathology of the parathyroid gland in hyperparathyroidism: study of twenty-five cases. Am. J. Path., 11:1, 1935.
——— and Mallory, T. B.: Parathyroid hyperplasia in chronic renal insufficiency. Ibid. 13:553, 1937.
Churchill, E. D.: The operative treatment of hyperparathyroidism. Ann. Surg., 100:606, 1934.
——— and Cope, O.: Parathyroid tumors associated with hyperparathyroidism. Surg., Gynec. & Obst., 58:255, 1934.
——— and Cope, O.: The surgical treatment of hyperparathyroidism. Ann. Surg., 104:9, 1936.
Collip, J. B., Clark, E. P., and Scott, J. W.: The effect of a parathyroid hormone on normal animals. J. Biol. Chem., 63:439, 1925.
———: The parathyroid glands. Medicine, 5:1, 1926.
Cope, O.: Surgery of hyperparathyroidism: the occurrence of parathyroids in the anterior mediastinum and the division of the operation into two stages. Ann. Surg., 114:706, 1941.
———: The endocrine aspects of enlargements of parathyroid glands. Surgery, 16:273, 1944.
———: The endocrine aspects of enlargements of the parathyroid glands; in Endocrinology of Neoplastic Diseases. New York, Oxford University Press, 1947, p. 338.
———: Hyperparathyroidism: 67 cases in ten years. J. Missouri M.A., 39:273, 1942.
Hannon, R. R., Shorr, E., McClellan, W. S., and DuBois, E. F.: A case of osteitis fibrosa cystica (osteomalacia?) with evidence of hyperactivity of the parathyroid bodies: metabolic study. J. Clin. Investigation, 8:215, 1930.
Ingalls, T. H., Donaldson, G. A., and Albright, F.: The locus of action of the parathyroid hormone: experimental studies with parathyroid extract on normal and nephrectomized rats. J. Clin. Investigation, 22:603, 1943.
Jaffe, H. L.: Primary and secondary (renal) hyperparathyroidism. S. Clin. North America, 22:621, 1942.

Keating, F. R., Jr., and Cook, E. N.: The recognition of primary hyperparathyroidism. J.A.M.A., *129*:994, 1945.

Mandl, F.: Klinisches und Experimentelles zur Frage der lokalisierten und generalisierten Ostitis fibrosa: B. Die generalisierte Form der Ostitis fibrosa. Arch. f. klin. Chir., *143*:245, 1926.

McLean, F. C., and Hastings, A. B.: Clinical estimation and significance of calcium-ion concentration in the blood. Am. J. M. Sc., *189*:601, 1935.

Meyer, K. A., Rosi, P. A., and Ragins, A. B.: Carcinoma of the parathyroid gland. Surgery, *6*:190, 1939.

Moehlig, R. C., and Abbott, H. L.: Carbohydrate metabolism in osteitis deformans or Paget's disease. J.A.M.A., *134*:1521, 1947.

Pappenheimer, A. M., and Wilens, S. L.: Enlargement of the parathyroid glands in renal disease. Am. J. Path., *11*:73, 1935.

Patt, H. M., Wallerstein, E., and Luckhardt, A. B.: A humoral control of parathyroid secretion. Proc. Soc. Exper. Biol. & Med., *49*:580, 1942.

Recklinghausen, F. von: Die fibröse oder deformirende Osteitis, die Osteomalacie und die osteoplastiche carcinose in ihren gegenseitigen Beziehungen. Festschrift Rudolph Virchow. Berlin, Reiner, 1891.

Riegel, C., Royster, H. P., Gislason, G. J., and Hughes, P. B.: Chemical studies in hyperparathyroidism and urolithiasis. J. Urol., *57*:192, 1947.

Rienhoff, W. F.: The surgical treatment of hyperparathyroidism. Ann. Surg., *131*:917, 1950.

Royster, H. P.: [Discussion of Rienhoff's paper, same issue.] Ann. Surg., *131*:943, 1950.

Tweedy, W. R., Chilcote, M. E., and Patras, M. C.: Distribution, retention and excretion of radiophosphorus following thyro-parathyroidectomy, or bilateral nephrectomy, and administration of parathyroid extract. J. Biol. Chem., *168*:597, 1947.

Walton, A. J.: Surgical treatment of parathyroid tumors. Brit. J. Surg., *19*:285, 1931.

Wellbrock, W. L. A.: Malignant adenoma of the parathyroid glands. Endocrinology, *13*:285, 1929.

Wilder, R. M., and Howell, L. P.: Etiology and diagnosis of hyperparathyroidism. A review of 135 proved cases. J.A.M.A., *106*:427, 1936.

CHAPTER 9

FUNCTIONING TUMORS OF THE ISLANDS OF LANGERHANS

HISTORICAL CONSIDERATIONS

The evolution of our knowledge of hyperinsulinism has been the result of many individual contributions. Perhaps the first time the pancreas was associated with diabetes was in 1788 when Cawley reported the autopsy findings of a diabetic patient who presented pancreatic calculi. In 1856 Claude Bernard wrote upon glycosuria and hyperglycemia with a discernment which advanced thought in this field. Thirteen years later, in 1869, Paul Langerhans, while still a medical student, wrote his medical thesis on the islands to which his name was subsequently affixed by Laguesse. The latter author suggested that this portion of the pancreatic tissue might have an endocrine function. In 1884 Arnozan and Vaillard ligated the ducts of the pancreas and noted an atrophy of the acinar tissue and a persistence of the islet cells. They failed, however, to attach significance to the persistence of the islet cells in an animal which did not develop diabetes. In 1889 von Mehring and Minkowski produced a fatal diabetes in animals by total pancreatectomy, and two years later Minkowski demonstrated that a successful graft of pancreatic tissue would prevent diabetes following total pancreatectomy, with diabetes ensuing when the graft was also excised. In 1895 Schafer noted the evidence in favor of an internal secretion of the pancreas by pointing out that, while total pancreatectomy produced a fatal diabetes, a total external pancreatic fistula did not. Opie, in 1901, described hyaline changes in the islet cells of diabetics at autopsy. Against this background Banting and Best, in 1922, isolated insulin and demonstrated its efficacy in the treatment of diabetes mellitus.

Shortly after the clinical picture of insulin overdosage began to be observed and appreciated, Harris noted similar symptoms in certain other patients with hypoglycemia and postulated in 1924 that hyperplasia or neoplasia of the islands of Langerhans must exist in such patients. Three years later such a case was studied by Wilder and his associates, and this patient, a physician suffering from the syndrome of severe insulin shock, was operated upon by W. J. Mayo. A tumor of the pancreas was found, with multiple liver metastases. A biopsy of the metastases revealed an islet cell carcinoma, and biologic assay on standardized rabbits revealed that the metastases contained insulin as shown by their ability to lower the blood sugar of these animals. The first case successfully treated surgically was operated upon by Graham of Toronto and was reported by Howland and his associates. At operation a benign adenoma of islet tissue was removed and the patient was cured.

PATHOLOGY OF ISLET CELL TUMORS

As intimated in the historical sketch, the pathologic physiology of excessive islet cell function is the result of the large amount of insulin released into the blood stream with the attendant hypoglycemia. Nicholls first described a tumor of the islands of Langerhans in 1902 but he gave

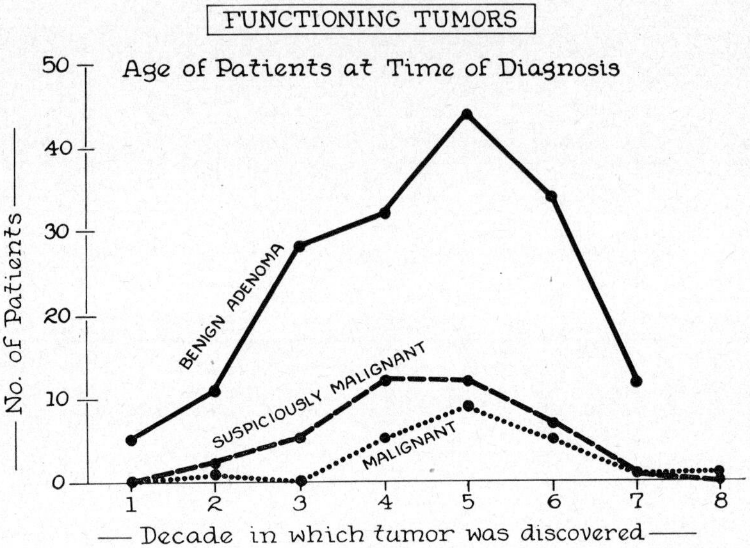

Fig. 35. Age distribution of functioning tumors of the pancreas. (Howard, J. M., Moss, N. H., and Rhoads, J. E.: Internat. Abstr. Surg., 90:426, 1950; in Surg., Gynec. & Obst., May 1950.)

no clinical history and thus, for practical purposes, it was not until the syndrome of insulin shock resulted in Harris's suggestion that hypertrophy or hyperplasia of the islands might explain certain types of spontaneous hypoglycemia seen clinically that physicians were prompted to search for this condition. Since that time surgeons have become widely familiar with these tumors. They are usually reddish brown in color and contrast with the yellow or ivory color of the surrounding pancreas. Moreover, they are of a firmer consistency and "feel like capsulated marbles to the palpating fingers" (Whipple).

These tumors, usually benign, well circumscribed and small (average diameter 1 to 2 cm.), are found more frequently in the tail or body of the pancreas, since islet tissue is more abundant in these areas. Nevertheless, one must also search carefully for nodules in the head of the pancreas, not only because the tumors may be multiple but because the adenomas in the head of the pancreas are the ones most frequently overlooked. Occasionally these tumors are large, and Braunschwig has removed one which measured 15 by 13 by 10 cm. Yet, this patient's symptoms were no more severe than those experienced by patients with smaller tumors.

Other types of pathology may be encountered in the islets. At times there may be present only a generalized hyperplasia of the pancreatic tissue, and occasionally an islet cell tumor may be malignant. The microscopic appearance of the benign adenoma is quite similar to that of normal islet tissue. Boyd suggests that a simple way to distinguish between tumor cells and the cells of the gland acini is to stain the zymogen granules of the latter, as this is much easier than to stain the specific granules of the tumor (islet) cells. Where there is blood vessel invasion it is often very difficult to be certain of the exact degree of malignancy. Frantz, in a careful follow-up study of ninety-one cases, found that twenty-one of these had originally been considered malignant. However, the follow-up results over a considerable period of time were so good that the author found it difficult to believe that all the twenty-one cases considered to be carcinoma were indeed malignant. In respect to this difficulty in evaluating the significance of blood vessel invasion, the islet cell tumor is similar to certain tumors of the thyroid whose malignancy is of a very low grade.

Finally, there are islet cell tumors, both benign and malignant, which do not secrete abnormal amounts of insulin.

THE DIAGNOSIS OF HYPERINSULINISM

The diagnosis of hyperinsulinism should be considered in any patient who presents the clinical picture elicited by hypoglycemia. Wilder has grouped the nervous components of this syndrome under three headings: those related to the vegetative nervous system, consisting of nausea, sweating, pallor, flushing, chilliness and syncope; those arising from the central nervous system, represented by restlessness, tonic or clonic muscle spasms, opisthotonos and convulsions; and psychic disturbances such as apprehension, disorientation, mania, confusion, unconsciousness and coma.

At times the "attacks" are represented by digestive disturbances and abdominal pain. In 1938 Whipple emphasized the following findings which he considered to represent an indispensable *diagnostic triad:* (1) The "attacks" come on characteristically in the early morning during the fasting period before breakfast, or following intensive mental or physical effort when sugar reserves are low; (2) during the "attacks" or after a prolonged fast of at least twelve hours the blood sugar levels are always below 50 mg. per 100 cc.; and (3) the patients recover promptly from the "spell," whatever their pattern may be, on the administration of sugar by mouth or by vein.

This triad has been generally accepted, and rigid adherence to its dicta has resulted in a gratifyingly high percentage of accurate preopera-

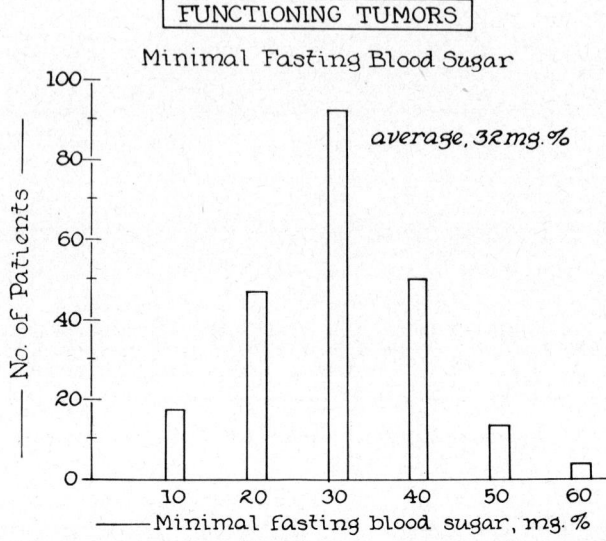

Fig. 36. Functioning tumors of the pancreas: minimal fasting blood sugar levels. (Howard, J. M., Moss, N. H., and Rhoads, J. E.: Internat. Abstr. Surg., 90:426, 1950; in Surg., Gynec. & Obst., May 1950.)

tive diagnoses. Whipple found a tumor in twenty-seven of twenty-eight cases in which a typical triad was present preoperatively.

Differential Diagnosis

A demonstrable tumor or hyperplasia of the pancreatic islets is of course not the only cause of hypoglycemia. The factors regulating glucose metabolism are many, and it may at times be exceedingly difficult, if not impossible, to arrive at an accurate diagnosis. Dysfunction of any of the following organs may affect glucose metabolism: the pituitary, adrenal cortex, adrenal medulla, thyroid gland, liver, and the hypothalamus. Womack has pointed out that the carbohydrate of the diet is not nearly so important in the maintenance of the blood sugar level as it was formerly thought to be.

In discussing the spontaneous hypoglycemias, Conn has suggested four principal categories: 1. *Organic hyperinsulinism,* in 75 per cent of which cases a tumor will be found at operation. Organic hyperinsulinism must be managed surgically. Conservative management with a high carbohydrate diet only leads to obesity, and the repeated attacks of hypoglycemia may result in cerebral damage. Moreover, there is ever present

FUNCTIONING TUMORS OF THE ISLANDS OF LANGHERHANS 115

the possibility of malignant changes in the adenoma. 2. *Functional hyperinsulinism,* wherein the insulin response to the dietary intake is excessive but not persistent. This type of hypoglycemia may be managed satisfactorily with appropriate diets. 3. *Hepatogenic hypoglycemia,* in which there is liver damage and a diminished glycogen reserve. Such a condition may be found in severe hyperthyroidism and here it is important to administer glucose to prevent hypoglycemia and to aid in liver repair. 4. *Pituitary* and *adrenal hypoglycemia,* and *renal glycosuria.*

SURGICAL MANAGEMENT OF ORGANIC HYPERINSULINISM

For adequate exposure of the pancreas a wide transverse incision just above the umbilicus is satisfactory. The gastrocolic omentum is divided

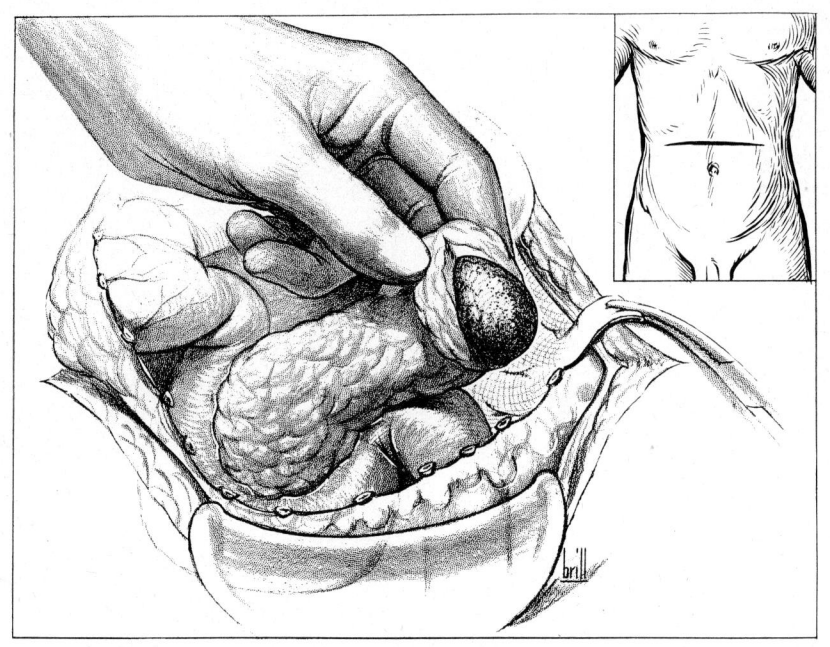

Fig. 37. Exposure of islet cell tumor of the pancreas.

and the entire pancreas is visualized. On the basis of his rich experience in dealing with islet adenomas, Whipple has suggested the following considerations. After "loading" the patient with a fortifying infusion of glucose the operation is begun with an anesthetic suited to the individual. Since the tumors are more likely to be found in the tail or body of the pancreas, these portions of the organ are examined first. If the anterior surface is normal, the peritoneal attachment along the inferior border should be divided and by careful blunt dissection the posterior surface should be elevated and inspected. If no reddish tumor is seen, the gland is carefully palpated for a marble-like nodule firmer than the remainder of the pancreatic tissue. If no tumor is seen or felt in the body or tail, the duodenum is reflected medially and the head of the pancreas carefully examined in the same way. While care must be exercised to avoid injury to the common duct, this consideration must be met with skill and the most thorough search carried out. If one tumor is found the search should be continued, since there are not infrequently present multiple adenomas. If no tumor is found, the feasibility of subtotal or total pancreatic resection must be considered. The results of subtotal resection have not been nearly so satisfactory as those following the successful removal of an adenoma. This has been due at times to an inadequate resection and in other instances to the failure to find an adenoma in the portion of the pancreas left behind. Indeed, so serious is the possibility of overlooking an adenoma which may ultimately prove fatal that Priestley and his associates at the Mayo Clinic performed a total pancreatectomy on one patient with an islet cell adenoma whose tumor could not be found at operation. This patient developed a relatively mild type of diabetes. Although a disturbance of carbohydrate digestion was not found, protein and fat digestion was impaired to the extent that 35 to 70 per cent of ingested fat and 25 to 55 per cent of ingested nitrogen could be found in the feces, and foodstuffs in the urine and feces accounted for 21 to 34 per cent of caloric intake. Nevertheless, a positive nitrogen balance was obtained.

In removal of the adenoma, bleeding is usually readily controlled with silk ligatures, which withstand the digestive properties of pancreatic juice. If radical subtotal pancreatectomy is contemplated, it is advantageous to remove the spleen also. Ligation of the splenic artery aids in controlling the arterial blood supply to the body and tail of the pancreas. The simple "shelling out" of an adenoma does not usually necessitate drainage, but the pancreatic bed should be drained with rubber dam or cigarette drains following resection of pancreatic tissue.

Postoperative Care. Although the other islets do not usually manifest the same degree of atrophy in the presence of a functioning adenoma as do the parathyroid glands, the patient may present a diabetic picture in the immediate postoperative period. A moderate hyperglycemia need cause little concern, but the development of frank acidosis should be prevented with appropriate insulin dosage.

Prognosis. The results are excellent when the adenomatous tissue is found and removed. These patients are cured. The results are much less satisfactory if no adenoma is found and a subtotal or total resection is performed. Usually either an adenoma in the head of the pancreas is overlooked or too little pancreas is resected. Total pancreatectomy is a radical procedure and does not leave the patient in a physiologic condition. The results are universally bad when a tumor with metastases is found.

Surgery should be advised immediately once the diagnosis of an islet cell adenoma has been made. This will prevent excessive obesity, it will prevent further mental deterioration from repeated "shocks," and there is an excellent chance that the adenoma will be successfully removed and the patient cured.

REFERENCES

Allan, F. N., and Marshall, S. F.: The surgical treatment of islet tumors of the pancreas with hyperinsulinism. S. Clin. North America, 25:719, 1945.

Arnozan, X., and Vaillard, L.: Contribution à l'étude du pancreas du lapin; lésions provoqués par la ligature du canal de Wirsung. Arch. de physiol. norm. et path., 3:287, 1884.

Banting, F. G., Best, C. H., and others: Pancreatic extracts in the treatment of diabetes mellitus. Canad. M. A. J., 12:141, 1922.

—— and Best, C. H.: Internal secretion of the pancreas. J. Lab. & Clin. Med., 7: 251, 1922.

Bernard, C.: Mémoire sur le pancréas et sur le rôle du suc pancréatique dans les phénomèns digestifs. Compt. rend Acad. d. sc. (Supp.), 1:379, 1856. (Quoted by Whipple, A. O.: Hyperinsulinism in relation to pancreatic tumors. Surgery, 16: 289, 1944.)

Boyd, W.: Surgical Pathology. 6th ed. Philadelphia, W. B. Saunders Company, 1947, p. 354.

Braunschwig, A.: The Surgery of Pancreatic Tumors. St. Louis, C. V. Mosby Co., 1942, p. 421.

Brush, B. A., and McClure, R. D.: Hyperinsulinism treated by subtotal pancreatectomy. Ann. Surg., 120:750, 1944.

Cawley, T.: A singular case of diabetes, consisting entirely in the quality of the urine. London M. J., 9:286, 1788.

Conn, J. W.: The spontaneous hypoglycemias. J.A.M.A., 115:1669, 1940.

Copp, E. F. F., and Barclay, A. J.: The restoration of hydropically degenerated cells of the pancreatic islands in dogs under insulin treatment. J. Metabolic Research, 4:445, 1923.

Cori, C. F., and Cori, G. T.: Carbohydrate metabolism. Ann. Rev. Biochem., 15:193, 1946.

David, V.: The indications and results of pancreatectomy for hypoglycemia. Surgery, 8:212, 1940.

Duff, G. L.: The pathology of islet cell tumors of the pancreas. Am. J. M. Sc., 203: 1437, 1942.

Frantz, V. K.: Tumors of the islet cells with hyperinsulinism; benign, malignant and questionable. Ann. Surg., 112:161, 1940.

Gomori, G.: Pathology of the pancreatic islets. Arch. Path., 36:217, 1943.

Graham, E. A., and Hartmann, A. F.: Subtotal resection of the pancreas in hypoglycemia. Surg., Gynec. & Obst., 59:474, 1934.

—— and Womack, N. A.: The application of surgery to the hypoglycemic state due to islet tumors of the pancreas and to other conditions. Surg., Gynec. & Obst., 56: 728, 1933.

Harris, S.: Gastrointestinal manifestations of hyperinsulinism. Am. J. Digest. Dis. & Nutrition, 2:557, 1935.

———: Hyperinsulinism and dysinulinism. J.A.M.A., 83:729, 1924.

Homans, J.: The study of experimental diabetes in the canine and its relation to human diabetes. J. M. Research, 33:1, 1915.

Houssay, B. A.: Hypophysis and metabolism (Dunham Lecture). New England J. Med., 214:961, 1936.

———: What we have learned from toad concerning hypophyseal functions (Dunham Lecture). Ibid., 913.

Howland, G., Campbell, W. R., Maltby, E. J., and Robinson, W. L.: Dysinulinism, convulsions and coma due to islet cell tumor of the pancreas with operation and cure. J.A.M.A., 93:674, 1929.

Laguesse, E.: Sur la formation des ilots de Langerhans dans les pancréas. Compt. rend. Soc. de biol., 45:819, 1893.

Laidlow, G. F.: Pathology of islet cell tumors. Am. J. Path., *14:*125, 1938.

Langerhans, P.: Beitrage zur mikroskopischen Anatomie der Bauchspeicheldruse. Berlin, Lange, 1869.

Long, C. N. H., and Lukens, F. D. W.: The effects of adrenalectomy and hypophysectomy upon experimental diabetes in the cat. J. Exper. Med., *63:*465, 1936.

Marble, A., and McKittrick, L. C.: Islet cell tumors of the pancreas with hyperinsulinism. New England J. Med., *235:*639, 1946.

Mehring, J. von, and Minkowski, O.: Diabetes mellitus nach Pankreasextirpation. Arch. f. exper. Path. u. Pharmakol., *26:*371, 1889.

Minkowski, O.: Untersuchungen über den Diabetes mellitus nach Extirpation des Pankreas. *Ibid.*, *31:*85, 1893.

Nicholls, A. G.: Simple adenoma of the pancreas arising from an island of Langerhans. J. M. Research, *8:*385, 1902.

O'Leary, J. L.: An experimental study of the islet cells of the pancreas in vivo. Anat. Rec., *45:*27, 1930.

——— and Womack, N. A.: Histology of adenoma of islets of Langerhans. Arch. Path., *17:*291, 1934.

Opie, E. L.: The relation of diabetes mellitus to lesions of the pancreas. J. Exper. Med., *5:*527, 1901.

Priestley, J. T., Comfort, M. W., and Radcliffe, J., Jr.: Total pancreatectomy for hyperinsulinism due to an islet cell adenoma: survival and cure at sixteen months after operation; presentation of metabolic studies. Ann. Surg., *119:*211, 1944.

Riffenburgh, R. S.: Islet cell adenoma of the pancreas. Am. Pract., *2:*276, 1947.

Schafer, E. A.: Internal secretions. Lancet, *2:*321, 1895.

Whipple, A. O.: Hyperinsulinism in relation to pancreas tumors; in Endocrinology of Neoplastic Diseases. New York, Oxford University Press, 1947, p. 357.

———: The surgical therapy of hyperinsulinism. J. internat. chir., *3:*237, 1938.

Wilder, R. M.: Hyperinsulinism (Colver Lecture). Internat. Clin., *2:*1, 1933.

———, Allan, F. N., Power, M. H., and Robertson, H. E.: Carcinoma of the islands of the pancreas; hyperinsulinism and hypoglycemia. J.A.M.A., *89:*348, 1927.

Womack, N. A.: Hypoglycemia. Surgery, *2:*793, 1937.

CHAPTER 10

THE ADRENAL GLANDS: SURGICAL CONSIDERATIONS

The pathologic lesions of the adrenal glands which are of particular interest to the surgeon are the cortical tumors, cortical hyperplasia and the medullary pheochromocytoma. There is also at present a considerable interest among both surgeons and internists in the possible relationship between adrenocortical activity and essential hypertension. Available data concerning the value of subtotal or total adrenalectomy in this connection will be mentioned.

ADRENAL CORTICAL TUMORS AND HYPERPLASIA

Clinical Manifestations. The clinical signs of hyperplasia of the adrenal cortex with associated hyperfunction vary widely. There are adenomas which produce no endocrine changes and which are discovered only as incidental findings at autopsy, but the majority of adrenal tumors are usually attended by fairly striking physical alterations. Kenyon has outlined in practical form these manifestations, grouped into the clinical patterns seen most frequently. His classification follows:

1. Adrenogenital syndrome: in children of either sex but more frequently in girls and occasionally in adult females. Masculinization may be intense.

2. Cushing's syndrome: in women and children. Masculinization is much less intense than in the adrenogenital syndrome and consists mostly of abnormalities in growth of hair. There may be a "buffalo" type of obesity, a plethoric appearance with a "moon-like" face, hypertension, purple striae, ecchymoses, osteoporosis and diabetes mellitus. Amenorrhea is usually present in women. This clinical picture may be associated with adrenocortical hyperplasia as well as with adrenocortical tumors, thymic tumors with adrenal hyperplasia, ovarian arrhenoblastoma, and pituitary tumors with or without adrenal hyperplasia.

3. Mixed clinical pictures including features of the first two categories. For instance, there may be hypertension, striae and glycosuria, individually or together, where intense masculinization is present.

4. A type characterized by single or isolated endocrine manifestations.

5. Feminizing syndromes, a rare manifestation in men characterized

120　SURGERY AND THE ENDOCRINE SYSTEM

by atrophy of the testis, loss of body hair, and growth of the breasts. Girls may show precocious breast enlargement and menstruation.

6. Tumors without endocrine function.

This classification is extremely helpful in utilizing our present knowledge in recognizing these varied manifestations as representative of adrenocortical dysfunction, but it is still inadequate to cover all the variations which one meets in association with tumors or hyperplasia of

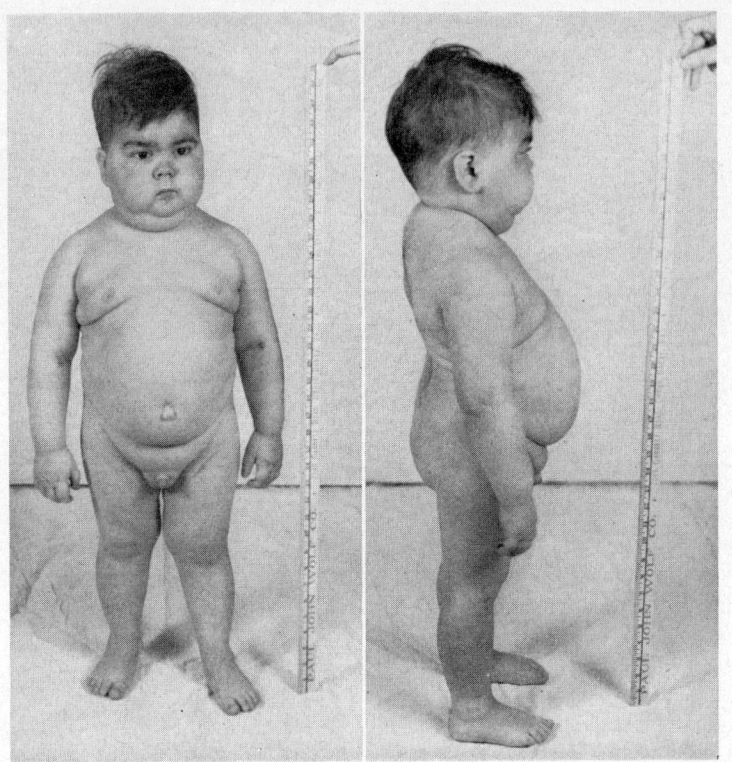

Fig. 38. Adrenocortical hyperplasia in two-year-old boy. (Courtesy Drs. E. K. Rose, E. Rose and J. E. Rhoads; to be published.)

the adrenal cortex. An approach which may ultimately replace empiric observations as a means of classifying adrenal tumors is the correlation of patterns of urinary steroid excretion with clinical pictures. The identity and action of the known steroids of the adrenal cortex have been considered briefly under the section on the response to stress, and only the quantitative aspects of total corticoid and total 17-ketosteroid excretion in the urine in cortical neoplasia will be mentioned here.

Outline of Diagnostic Procedures for Adrenocortical Tumors

History. Any suggestion of abnormal sexual development, unusual fat distribution, striae, etc.

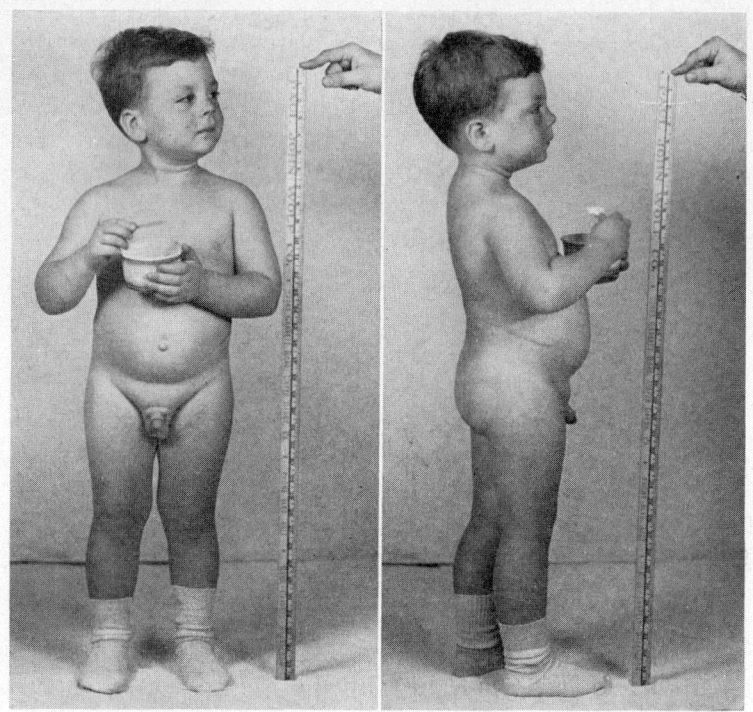

THE ADRENAL GLANDS: SURGICAL CONSIDERATIONS 121

Fig. 39. Patient shown in Figure 38, five months after resection of four-fifths of each adrenal. (Courtesy of Drs. E. K. Rose, E. Rose and J. E. Rhoads.)

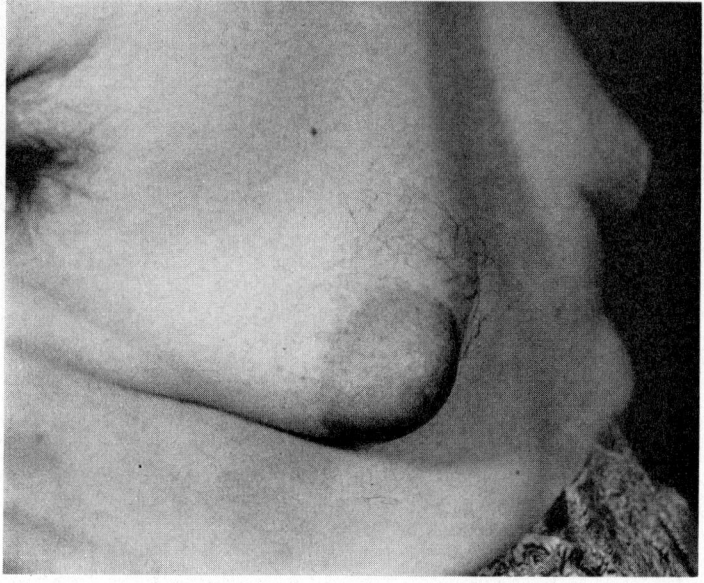

Fig. 40. Feminizing tumor of adrenal cortex with resulting gynecomastia in a middle-aged male. (Courtesy of Dr. Wallace W. Dyer.)

Physical Examination. Careful search for any signs listed above under clinical manifestations. A mass may be palpable.

Blood Chemistry. *Serum Chloride, Carbon Dioxide, Potassium, Sodium.* Abnormalities may vary, depending upon preponderance of certain corticoids (steroid compounds with 21 carbon atoms).

Fasting Blood Sugar and Glucose Tolerance Curve. Occasionally tumors may produce a picture simulating diabetes mellitus.

Urinary Studies. *The Colorimetric Assay of Urinary Corticoid-like Substances (11-Oxysteroids).* Talbot and his associates consider the normal range to lie between 0.17 and 0.34 mg. per twenty-four hours. However, the results obtained by other methods may be somewhat higher, and normal controls must be run by each laboratory. Marked increases may be observed in adrenocortical neoplasia, Cushing's syndrome, severe burns and other trauma.

Colorimetric Determination of the Urinary Excretion of 17-Ketosteroids per Twenty-four Hours. Normal adult women excrete from 5 to 17 mg. of 17-ketosteroids per twenty-four hours, with an average excretion of about 10 mg. Normal men excrete from 6 to 25 mg., with an average excretion of about 14 mg. The excretion may be markedly elevated in Cushing's syndrome. Values above 50 mg. are suggestive and values above 100 mg. are usually diagnostic of adrenocortical hyperfunction. The 17-ketosteroid excretion is diminished in the aged, the malnourished, in myxedema, in chronic stress states, including starvation, and in acute and chronic liver disease.

Roentgenologic Examinations. *Plain Flat Plate of Abdomen.* Obviously the tumor of the adrenal must be large to be visible on such a film and, unfortunately, most such tumors are not this large. Body section films may be useful.

Intravenous Urogram and Retrograde Pyelogram. These procedures may reveal displacement of the kidney on the side where the tumor is located.

Perirenal Air Injection. Cahill has reported a considerable experience with this method and he considers it more dependable, though more hazardous, than urography. We have not used this method since a fatality which occurred a number of years ago. Walters and Sprague have recently written of perirenal air injection: "Moreover, in a few cases in which we injected air, the reaction was rather shocking both to the patient and to us, so that we abandoned this method of diagnosis, not because of this alone, but also because of the ease, safety and accuracy with which the adrenal glands can be exposed through a small surgical incision."

Search for Bone Age and Premature Closure of Epiphyses (Under Age Twenty-one); Osteoporosis (if with Cushing's Syndrome).

Examination of the Chest for Metastases. Many of the adrenocortical tumors are malignant.

Films to Rule Out Lesions Other Than Adrenal. (*a*) Pituitary fossa for possible pituitary tumor; (*b*) signs of increased intracranial pressure; (*c*) ventriculograms, where indicated; (*d*) possible increased calcification and displacement of the pineal gland; (*e*) search for mediastinal enlargement, since a thymic tumor may rarely be associated with Cushing's syndrome.

Surgical Exploration. Occasionally it may be impossible, on the basis of the studies listed above, to reach a conclusive diagnosis as to whether or not the site of disease is the pituitary fossa, pineal gland, floor of the fourth ventricle, thymus, adrenals or ovaries. Even if the pituitary fossa were freed from suspicion and all other sites except the ovaries and adrenals excluded, it might be impossible to make the differential diagnosis between an adrenal lesion and a masculinizing tumor of the ovary. Under these circumstances an exploratory laparotomy may be required. If this is done, many surgeons consider it wise actually to take a biopsy of ovarian tissue, rather than to rely upon mere visual inspection and palpation. Examination of the adrenals may be carried out at the same time or at a subsequent operation.

Preoperative Preparations and Postoperative Care

The patient with a hyperfunctioning adrenocortical tumor on one side may have sustained a considerable atrophy of the adrenal cortex on the opposite side. This is the basis of the substantial operative mortality reported following excision of these tumors in the past. Very rarely, there may be no adrenal on the opposite side (Lukens and others). Cahill has stated that acute adrenal insufficiency occurs only or mostly in those patients with symptoms described as Cushing's syndrome and which are due to an excessive secretion of corticoids (C-21 steroids). The symptoms which herald the approach of acute adrenal insufficiency in the postoperative period are marked anorexia, hiccough, nausea, vomiting, insomnia, apathy, disorientation, restlessness, weakness and apprehension. The signs are an increased pulse rate, a fall in blood pressure, and a rise in temperature. Of these, we have found the fall in blood pressure and the rise in temperature especially significant. A marked anorexia has also been a prominent feature in our patients. Of the laboratory determinations, a rise in the blood urea nitrogen concentration has proved a far more sensitive indicator of approaching crisis than have changes in the serum chloride, sodium and potassium values. This has been particularly true in the early postoperative period. If acute adrenocortical insufficiency is to occur following the removal of a tumor of the adrenal cortex, it will usually develop within the first seventy-two hours following operation.

The availability of cortisone has greatly simplified the postoperative management of these patients. Formerly treatment consisted of the preoperative administration of 30 to 50 cc. of adrenocortical extract the night before operation and again immediately preoperatively. Another 50 cc. of cortical extract were given postoperatively and this dosage was repeated each day for several days. Saline and glucose were administered and desoxycorticosterone acetate, given intramuscularly, was also helpful. These measures are still of great value, but the liberal administration of cortisone preoperatively and postoperatively has largely eliminated the hazard of acute postoperative adrenal insufficiency. In addition, the administration of 25 to 50 mg. of ACTH every six hours for four to five days preceding operation may utilize the secretory capacity of the adrenocortical tumor to saturate the body tissues with a reserve supply of adrenocortical steroids for the immediate postoperative period. Cortisone has been administered either intramuscularly or by mouth with good effect by each route, and an intravenous preparation is now available. We have administered doses of the order of 10 to 25 mg. each six hours during the first forty-eight hours postoperatively, followed by the same dosage every twelve hours until, on the basis of clinical and laboratory evaluation, the patient was considered out of danger. Larger doses have been given when required, and intravenous saline, glucose and blood have been used freely. Although cortisone does not encompass the entire physiologic action of whole adrenocortical extract in all instances, it apparently substitutes effectively for the more important of these effects and, supplemented with small amounts (10 mg.) of DOCA, it has proved invaluable in the management of adrenocortical insufficiency.

Considerations in Technical Management
Surgical Exposure

Three general routes of approach for the resection of adrenal tumors have been used: (1) the "kidney" incision, extraperitoneally through the

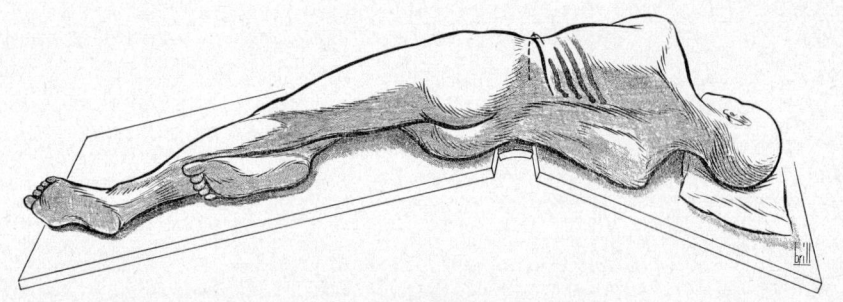

Fig. 41. Position of patient on table and location of incision for adrenalectomy. The table may be "broken" further if desired.

lumbar region; (2) transthoracically through the diaphragm; and (3) transperitoneally through the anterior abdominal wall. Each method has its advocates and obviously each has proved satisfactory in the hands of those who recommend it. Our opinion is that the transthoracic route

THE ADRENAL GLANDS: SURGICAL CONSIDERATIONS 125

gives good exposure but will usually require the resection of one rib with the probable division of another. This incision is likely to be more painful over a longer period of time. Furthermore, in addition to complications such as atelectasis, pneumothorax and empyema, which are to be considered possibilities following any thoracotomy, one exposes an additional serous cavity to possible contamination with tumor cells if the adrenal tumor proves malignant.

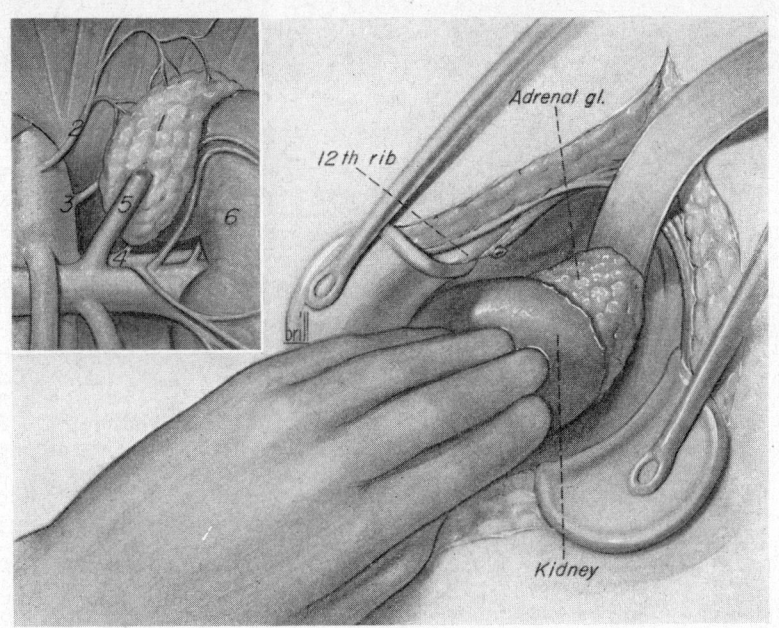

Fig. 42. Exposure of adrenal gland, and inset showing adrenal blood supply. *Inset:* 1. Adrenal gland. 2. Superior adrenal artery. 3. Middle adrenal artery. 4. Renal artery and inferior adrenal artery. 5. Adrenal vein. 6. Kidney. This arrangement of the adrenal vasculature is a very common one but it is not constant. For example, instead of one large vein emerging from the substance of the gland the vein may skirt the medial border of the adrenal, receiving several contributory vessels from within the gland. It is helpful in exposing the gland to remember that it occupies a more or less anterior position with respect to the upper pole of the kidney. *Below:* The capsule and fat of the kidney have been omitted for clarity, but we suggest that the renal capsule be left intact. If the kidney is retracted downward, the yellowish adrenal above it is readily distinguished from the less vivid surrounding fat.

The abdominal approach has much to recommend it if the tumor is large, and we have not hesitated to use it. However, in general we have preferred to use the lumbar or "kidney" incision, feeling that exposure was adequate and that contamination of the peritoneal cavity was thus avoided. Only on rare occasions has it been necessary to resect the twelfth rib.

Whenever it is possible to determine preoperatively the location of the tumor, that side should be explored first. It was formerly considered essential to determine if there were a second adrenal present on the opposite side, but the rarity with which one adrenal is absent and the present availability of supportive therapy for oral use at moderate cost (cortisone) render it the treatment of choice to remove the possibly malignant adrenocortical tumor in toto without regard to the presence or absence of the opposite adrenal.

Anatomical Features and Landmarks

The two adrenal glands sit astride the upper poles of the kidneys, the convex surfaces of the kidneys producing a concave impression on the glands. The right adrenal is somewhat more triangular than the left, its anterior surface touching the inferior vena cava posteriorly and medially and the liver laterally. The left adrenal is more crescentic in outline, lies along the anterior medial border of the left kidney, and its lower half is in contact anteriorly with the posterior surface of the pancreatic and splenic vessels. The left adrenal is nearer the aorta than is the right, and it lies behind the lesser omental sac. Both glands are situated in the epigastric region at the level of the eleventh thoracic vertebra and their posterior surfaces rest against the lumbar insertion of the diaphragmatic leaves.

The adrenals have a rich blood supply. The superior, middle and inferior arteries, which are branches of the inferior diaphragmatic artery, aorta and renal artery, respectively, penetrate into the gland to supply the cortex and medulla separately. On the right side venous drainage is usually into the vena cava and on the left into the renal vein.

The lymphatics of the right adrenal drain into the lymph nodes near the aorta and near the crus of the diaphragm. On the left side they connect with a node situated at the origin of the renal artery and with nodes between the aorta and the crus of the diaphragm (Soffer).

The innervation of the adrenals is chiefly by branches of the splanchnic nerves. These nerves then form the suprarenal plexus and connect with the renal and celiac plexuses and with the celiac ganglia.

The size and weight of the adrenals may vary greatly in various states of pathologic physiology, but the average weight of each adrenal is approximately 5 gm. The usual ranges of other dimensions are as follows: height, 3 to 5 cm.; breadth, 2.5 to 3 cm.; and thickness, approximately 0.2 to 0.8 cm., the organ being somewhat thicker at its base. The cut surface of the gland presents an outer cortical substance which is firm and yellowish owing to the lipid contained within the cells. There is an inner layer, the medulla, whose substance is softer, more pulpy, and of a dark reddish brown hue. The medulla comprises only about 10 per cent of the entire gland (Soffer).

The trabeculae from the capsule penetrate into the gland and form septa which divide the cortex into its three characteristic zones, the zona glomerulosa, the zona fasciculata, and the zona reticularis. There is evidence to suggest that these zones may prove to have different secretory activities.

Course to Follow After Exposure of the Adrenal

The decision as to how much adrenal tissue to remove can be an exceedingly dfficult one. We have reached the following tentative conclusions. If a tumor is found in the first adrenal exposed, this gland should be resected in its entirety. As stated previously, the chances that the tumor is malignant are considerable. Unfortunately, when these tumors are malignant they are apt to spread early and widely to the liver, lungs, brain and elsewhere. If a tumor is not found on the first side explored, the opposite adrenal is investigated. Bilateral nonmalignant adrenocortical tumors, unlike the pheochromocytoma of the medulla, are quite rare.

If hyperplasia of the adrenal gland associated with Cushing's syndrome is found, we have resected approximately three-quarters of the first adrenal and then exposed the second adrenal and resected approximately four-fifths of it. Resecting a major portion of the first adrenal before exposing the second is not as risky as it would seem at first thought, since if there were a functioning cortical tumor on the opposite side the first gland would usually be atrophic, in which case no tissue would be removed. Walters has advised preliminary exposure of both adrenals with partial resection of about three-fourths of only one gland at the first operation. If this should prove inadequate, he re-explores to determine the viability of the remnant of the previously resected gland, and, if it is viable, all or most of the gland on the opposite side is removed. This type of procedure has, to be sure, the real merit of an added margin of safety, lest too much adrenal tissue be removed. However, we feel that the availability of cortisone has materially diminished the hazard of removing too much adrenal tissue.

To recapitulate, the surgical management of an adrenocortical tumor is to resect the involved gland completely. The surgical management of bilateral cortical hyperplasia is still in the process of development and no final conclusions can be presented. Many surgeons in this field have advised subtotal resection of both glands when bilateral hyperplasia associated with Cushing's syndrome is encountered. It seems fair to say that the availability and ease of administration of oral cortisone will greatly modify our entire approach to the resection of adrenal tissue.

Prognosis Following Surgical Resection of Adrenocortical Tumors and Hyperplasia

The results to be expected following resection of cortical tumors may be summarized thus:

1. Removal of the tumor, if it is a single functioning adenoma, will

cure the syndrome, but often certain fixed changes may persist (e.g., bass voice in women). Removal of a functioning carcinoma may temporarily improve the patient, but the prognosis of this type of malignancy is poor.

2. In adrenal hyperplasia associated with Cushing's syndrome, subtotal resection of adrenal tissue may result in a temporary and at times quite prolonged disappearance of symptoms. However, neither the fundamental pathology nor the surgical course to be followed in this condition has been satisfactorily established. For this reason it is not possible to predict what the outcome of the individual case will be.

ADRENALECTOMY FOR ESSENTIAL HYPERTENSION

Dissatisfied with thoracolumbar sympathectomy as a means of therapy in many cases of severe essential hypertension, teams in a number of clinics have undertaken a comprehensive investigation of the value of subtotal and total adrenalectomy as a treatment for this disease. For details of background and management the reader is referred to the previous paragraphs on the preoperative and postoperative care of patients with adrenocortical tumors and to the publications of Green and his associates and of Zintel and his coworkers. Thorn, at the Peter Bent Brigham Hospital, has had an especially rich experience with these patients.

Dr. Zintel has permitted the following summary of the experience to date of his group at the Hospital of the University of Pennsylvania: "In a limited follow-up (roughly 12 months) it appears that subtotal adrenalectomy will produce some beneficial effects on the objective and subjective signs and symptoms as well as a variable reduction in the blood pressue of hypertensive patients. The possibility that subtotal adrenalectomy may find its greatest usefulness as an adjunct to limited or extensive sympathectomy and splanchnicectomy is being studied."

FUNCTIONING TUMORS OF THE ADRENAL MEDULLA (PHEOCHROMOCYTOMA)

Although certain characteristics of pheochromcytomas had been related by Manasse and others as early as 1893, it was not until 1922 that Labé, Tinel and Doumer recorded the first complete study of a classic case. They published a report of a young woman of twenty-eight who suffered from violent attacks of vomiting associated with tremor, chilliness and palpitation. Usually elevated, the blood pressure was highly variable. The patient died of acute pulmonary edema, and autopsy revealed a pheochromocytoma just above the left adrenal gland.

The first case of paroxysmal hypertension diagnosed during life was reported by Vaquez, Donzelot and Gerandel in 1926. Their patient was a man, aged thirty-seven, who experienced daily, most striking attacks of paroxysmal hypertension associated with severe cramps in the extremities, abdominal colic and violent headache. One such attack was attended by pulmonary edema and an intra-ocular hemorrhage which destroyed the vision of one eye. The patient left Vaquez and came under the care of Laubry who, knowing of the earlier diagnosis, treated him with deep roentgenotherapy over both adrenals. This therapy was effective in abolishing the attacks, at least up to the time of Laubry's report six months later.

In 1927 C. H. Mayo explored the abdomen of a woman, aged thirty, who had attacks of paroxysmal hypertension associated with dyspnea, headache, tachycardia and vomiting. A tumor intimately associated with the left adrenal was removed, and the patient was cured. On the basis of Mayo's experience, in 1929 Pincoffs was able to diagnose preoperatively a pheochromocytoma which was successfully removed and the patient cured. In 1937 Beer, King and Prinzmetal demonstrated preoperatively in an animal preparation a pressor substance in the patient's blood during crises. Following operation this effect was abolished.

Pathology of Pheochromocytomas

The pheochromocytoma is formed by chromaffin cells which are derived from the neuroectoderm of the neural crest, and these cells are developmentally related to the cells of the sympathetic ganglia. The pheochromocytoma has been described as histologically benign but physiologically malignant, since these tumors usually do not metastasize but eventually cause the death of the patient by the pathologic physiological changes resulting from the large amounts of epinephrine which they secrete into the blood stream. These tumors are usually small, round, encapsulated and unilateral. However, sixteen of 152 cases reported by MacKeith were bilateral. Whereas these tumors are usually in the adrenal glands or near by in the retroperitoneal space (Ganem and Cahill), they may be found elsewhere in the body and may even be intrathoracic (Maier; Phillips). If the tumor is malignant the metastases are to the regional lymph nodes, liver and skeleton. Large tumors are frequently necrotic and hemorrhagic, and the granules in the tumor cells give a characteristic brown chromaffin reaction when stained with chromium salts. Assays for epinephrine have varied from 0.12 to 20 mg. per gram of tumor tissue (Belt and Powell). The normal adrenal medulla contains only about 0.4 mg. of epinephrine per gram of tissue. Recently Goldenberg and his associates have used the paper chromatography technic to demonstrate the presence of norepinephrine in the adrenal medulla.

The pheochromocytoma is not a common tumor, but it is by no means rare. Over 200 cases have now been reported in the literature. Like the parathyroid adenomas, it seems probable that many cases of this condition are currently being overlooked or misdiagnosed. Of four cases reported by Bartels and Cattell from the Lahey Clinic, two had previously been diagnosed as hyperthyroidism and subjected to subtotal thyroidectomy elsewhere and a third had been referred to the clinic for thyroidectomy.

Clinical Picture

The clinical pictures presented by patients with pheochromocytoma may be of three general types: (1) the "typical attacks" associated with a paroxysmal hypertension; (2) chronic hypertension with renal and heart failure; and (3) no symptoms. MacKeith lists a fourth, Addison's disease from local pressure of the medullary tumor on the cortex, but surely this must be rare.

The history of the attacks may date back a number of years, and the initial attacks may have been mild. Although about one-half of the attacks are spontaneous, many patients are aware of precipitating factors such as postural changes (the most common), emotional or physical stress, pain, constipation and menstruation (Hatch, Richards and Spiegl).

Nature of the Paroxysmal Attacks. The paroxysmal attacks or "crises" so commonly associated with pheochromocytomas are the result of the liberation of excessive amounts of epinephrine into the blood stream. The symptoms experienced are palpitation, precordial sensations, nausea, vomiting, dizziness, pallor, coldness of the extremities, glycosuria, headache and anxiety. At the height of an attack the pupils may be dilated and pulmonary edema may intervene, a condition which not infrequently is a major contributing cause of death in such patients. During these episodes, which may last from a few minutes to days (average one to two hours), the blood pressure is usually markedly elevated above normal levels, only to fall again between paroxysms. However, if the disease persists long enough the blood pressure may become chronically elevated, and in such cases it may prove most difficult to exclude other causes of hypertension. Indeed, Green has drawn a forceful parallel between the chronic stages of essential hypertension and the hypertension caused by a pheochromocytoma. However, he is careful to point out that the angiospastic substance in essential hypertension is not necessarily epinephrine. Prohaska, Harms and Dragstedt, on the basis of experiments dealing with sustained hypertension of two weeks' duration produced in dogs with intravenous epinephrine, concluded that essential hypertension in man is probably not due to an increase in the secretion of adrenalin. The modes of death in cases of untreated pheochromocytoma are acute pulmonary edema with shock and collapse during crises, cerebral hemorrhage, or chronic renal and cardiac failure.

At times the clinical picture, particularly the hypermetabolism and markedly elevated basal metabolic rate, may lead to an erroneous diagnosis of hyperthyroidism, and such patients have been subjected to thyroidectomy (Bartels and Cattell; McCullagh and Engel). Moreover, the disappearance of "diabetes mellitus" following resection of a pheochromocytoma has been reported by Duncan, Seamans and Howard. Thus, when

THE ADRENAL GLANDS: SURGICAL CONSIDERATIONS 131

diabetes, hypertension and hypermetabolism are encountered in the same patient one must list pheochromocytoma high among the diagnostic possibilities. Needless to say, every effort must be made to exclude other causes of hypertension.

Diagnostic Procedures

Physical Examination. An abdominal mass may be palpable in the flank. If on massage a typical attack is induced, the diagnosis of pheochromocytoma is virtually certain. If a tumor is not palpable, massage of the abdominal wall may still precipitate an attack, but the tumor is not necessarily present on the side massaged.

Roentgenologic Procedures. These should be directed toward visualization of the kidney area. A mass in the chest film may be the offending pheochromocytoma. (See also under adrenocortical tumors.)

Laboratory Studies Which May be Helpful. *Fasting Blood Sugar.* An increased blood sugar level may result from the action of epinephrine.

Glucose Tolerance Test. There may be a decreased tolerance associated with an otherwise impaired carbohydrate metabolism, but more frequently the curve is normal.

Basal Metabolic Rate. This may be greatly increased in the cases of pheochromocytoma, but other causes of an increased BMR must be excluded.

Urinary 17-Ketosteroid and Total Corticoid Excretion. The excretion of these products is often normal, but it may be increased. It is possible that the presence of an excessive amount of epinephrine for the stimulation of an increased release of ACTH from the pituitary is more than offset by a decreased amount of functional adrenocortical tissue, a result of encroachment on the cortex of the involved adrenal gland by the medullary tumor.

Demonstration of a Pressor Substance in the Patient's Blood During an Attack.

Specific Diagnostic Chemical Tests. Histamine, Mecholyl, tetraethylammonium bromide, Dibenamine and benzodioxane derivatives.

Specific Chemical Tests

In 1933 Fourneau and Bovet published the first work on the use of benzodioxane compounds as "sympathicolytique" agents. Since that time a number of these compounds, as well as other chemical agents, have received consideration as tests in the diagnosis of pheochromocytoma. These tests will be presented briefly.

Histamine Test (Roth and Kvale). The patient is given 0.05 mg. of histamine base intravenously. In normal subjects, hyper-reactors, and patients with essential hypertension the reaction is about equal to that resulting from the cold pressor test. However, the patients with essential hypertension may show circumoral pallor and experience headaches. In patients with pheochromocytoma, attacks may be precipitated within two minutes, consisting of severe headache, distress in the abdomen and later in the chest, groaning, restlessness, anxiety, circumoral pallor and excessive sweating associated with a marked rise in blood pressure. The test is not specific for pheochromocytoma, however, since histamine may fail to produce an attack (Bartels and Cattell).

Dibenamine (Spear and Griswold). Here the drug is slowly administered intravenously and its effect on a sustained hypertension is noted. Over periods up to one hour or more, following the administration of up to 200 mg. of the drug, the hypertension of the pheochromocytoma may fall to much lower levels. Spear and Griswold consider this strong evidence for such a tumor.

Mecholyl (Guarneri and Evans). This test is based upon the reaction to 25 mg. of the drug given subcutaneously. An initial fall in blood pressure of short duration, which is followed by a marked and more sustained rise to hypertensive levels, constitutes a positive test. Of twenty-seven controls studied by Guarneri and Evans, none showed the hypertensive reactor response. False positives with this test are few, but a failure of response does not rule out the presence of pheochromocytoma.

Tetraethylammonium Bromide ("Etamon") (LaDue, Murison and Pack). As with histamine and Mecholyl, Etamon is not a specific incitatory agent in the presence of pheochromocytoma, and a negative test does not exclude a tumor. (The chloride salt is now preferred.)

Benzodioxane Drugs (Goldenberg, Snyder and Aranow). There are a number of these compounds which have a lytic effect on epinephrine. An examination of the structural formulas of the benzodioxanes clarifies understanding of their pharmacologic action. The simplest aromatic sympathomimetic amine is phenylethylamine. The introduction of an oxygen atom between the side chain and the ring results in a compound with adrenolytic properties.

Phenylethylamine

Piperidylmethyl benzodioxane
(933F)

In addition to the compound designated 933F, there are at least two similar ones (1164F and 1071F) which have been used clinically. The basis of their use for the diagnosis of pheochromocytoma is that in nontoxic dosage their action is adrenolytic rather than sympatholytic. In the case of 933F, the test is performed in the following manner. Using approximately 10 mg. per square meter of body surface area with the unsedated, rested patient in a reclining position, an intravenous drip of saline is begun. After several control blood pressure readings the drug is administered through the intravenous needle over a two-minute period.

In the presence of pheochromocytoma, the attendant increase in circulating epinephrine is counteracted and a fall in blood pressure results. In hypertension from other causes a minimal effect, no effect, or a purely pressor response is produced. Normal subjects usually respond with a mild pressor response. The duration of the drug action is usually less than fifteen minutes. Though Drill has reported alarming hypertensive reactions in some patients who did not have a pheochromocytoma, at the Hospital of the University of Pennsylvania benzodioxane derivatives have been used in the diagnosis and management of these tumors with considerable success, and without serious unfavorable reactions.

Surgical Technic and Management

A good basal anesthetic is most helpful in avoiding emotional reactions which may precipitate an attack. We prefer a general anesthetic mixture. Relaxation is often better with spinal anesthesia, but the blood pressure may be more difficult to control. Since a hypertensive reaction may be anticipated at any time before the tumor is removed, a slow intravenous drip of saline solution should be started as soon as the patient is prepared for the operation to permit the administration of dibenamine or benzodioxane as needed to prevent the blood pressure from reaching dangerously high levels. Other than this, intravenous fluids should be kept to a minimum.

The surgical approaches to the adrenal glands have been described in the section on adrenocortical tumors. We have usually employed the "kidney" incision for the removal of pheochromocytomas, but if the tumor is large the abdominal approach is preferred. The exposure of the adrenal is facilitated if exposure of the kidney is avoided.

In 10 per cent of cases these tumors are bilateral, but we have not routinely exposed the second adrenal if the tumor was found on the first side examined. However, if the hypertension persists following resection of a tumor on the first side one should not hesitate to explore the other adrenal at a second procedure. (Bartels and Cattell explore both adrenals at the first operation.) As noted previously, the gland on the side opposite the tumor does not undergo atrophy in the presence of a pheochromocytoma, which is contrary to the situation obtaining with cortical tumors. Thus, while cortical tissue should be preserved where possible, resection of one entire gland is not as serious as with cortical tumors. If there is any question of malignancy, the entire gland should be removed.

The tumor should be exposed, delivered and resected with a minimum of trauma in order to avoid the release of excessive amounts of epinephrine. If possible, the vessels are exposed and clamped as a first objective. It is advisable to administer one of the adrenolytic drugs intravenously before or at the time of manipulation of the tumor. The amount of drug used preoperatively for diagnosis can usually be repeated with safety. Grimson and his associates have reported the use of a benzodioxane compound throughout the operation without significant changes in blood pressure.

Following resection of the tumor there may be a sudden fall in the blood pressure to shock levels. If this occurs, putting the patient in the Trendelenburg position may be all that is required. This was formerly thought to be due to a sudden lowering of the high level of circulating epinephrine to which the body had become accustomed, but since, as pointed out by Bartels and Cattell, this collapse state may occur while the pheochromocytoma is still in situ, it would seem that an excess of epinephrine, rather than a lack of it, is the cause of the shock and that the collapse is due to acute failure of the left side of the heart. This view is further supported by the report of Grimson and his coworkers on the beneficial effect of benzodioxane used throughout the operation to neutralize excessive amounts of circulating epinephrine. However, it must be recognized that many able surgeons still consider the collapse to be due to a lack of epinephrine. Thus, if all else fails, epinephrine should probably be administered. Happily, this question should soon be settled by additional experience with the use of adrenolytic drugs. A moderate hypotension may persist for several hours after operation without ill effect.

Other Adjuncts to Postoperative Supportive Therapy

Some students in this field have considered the postoperative hypotension to be due in part to an absolute or relative adrenocortical insufficiency and have advocated the administration of cortical extract, desoxycorticosterone and salt solution (Biskind, Meyer and Beadner).

Prognosis Following Surgery

If all the neoplastic tissue has been removed and it is not malignant, the patient will be cured. Poor results are due to deaths from collapse on the operating table or in the immediate postoperative period (these are rapidly decreasing in number), malignancy, remaining functioning tumor tissue that has been overlooked, or to the fact that irreversible vascular changes have already occurred at the time of operation.

REFERENCES

Bartels, E. C., and Cattell, R. B.: Pheochromocytoma: its diagnosis and treatment. Ann. Surg., *131*:903, 1950.
Beer, E., King, F. N., and Prinzmetal, M.: Pheochromocytoma with demonstration of pressor (adrenalin) substance in the blood preoperatively during hypertensive crises. *Ibid.*, *106*:85, 1937.
Belt, A. E., and Powell, T. O.: Clinical manifestations of the chromaffin cell tumors arising from the suprarenal medulla. Surg., Gynec. & Obst., *59*:9, 1934.
Biskind, G. R., Meyer, M. A., and Beadner, S. A.: Adrenal medullary tumor; pheochromocytoma cured by surgical intervention; clinical management, analysis of all reported cases. J. Clin. Endocrinology, *1*:113, 1941.
Brunschwig, A., Humphreys, E., and Roome, N.: The relief of paroxysmal hypertension by excision of pheochromocytoma. Surgery, *4*:361, 1938.

Cahill, G. F.: Air injections to demonstrate the adrenals by x-ray. J. Urol., *34*:238, 1935.
———: Hormonal tumors of the adrenal; in Endocrinology of Neoplastic Diseases. New York, Oxford University Press, 1947, p. 291.
———: Hormonal tumors of the adrenal. Surgery, *16*:233, 1944.
———, Melicou, M. M., and Darby, H. H.: Adrenal cortical tumors, the types of non-hormonal and hormonal tumors. Surg., Gynec. & Obst., *74*:281, 1942.
Calkings, E., and Howard, J. E.: Pheochromocytomas. J. Clin. Endocrinol., *7*:475, 1947.
Callow, N. H., Callow, R. K., and Emmens, C. W.: Calorimetric determination of substances containing the grouping CH_2CO in urine extracts and as an indication of androgen content. Biochem. J., *32*:1312, 1938.
Cushing, H.: Basophil adenomas of pituitary body and their clinical manifestations (pituitary basophilism). Bull. Johns Hopkins Hosp., *50*:137, 1932.
Dorfman, R. I., Potts, A. M., and Feil, M. L.: Studies on the bioassay of hormones; the use of radiosodium for the detection of small quantities of desoxycorticosterone. Endocrinology, *41*:464, 1947.
Drill, V. A.: Reaction from the use of benzodioxane (933F) in diagnosis of pheochromocytoma. New England J. Med., *241*:777, 1949.
Duncan, L. E., Jr., Semans, J. H., and Howard, J. E.: Adrenal medullary tumor (pheochromocytoma) and diabetes mellitus; disappearance of diabetes after removal of the tumor. Ann. Int. Med., *20*:815, 1944.
Engstrom, W. W.: Nature and significance of neutral steroids in human urine in normal and in abnormal states, with a preliminary consideration of the adrenal and gonadal steroids and the factors which influence their secretion and biological action. Yale J. Biol. & Med., *21*:21, 1948.
Fourneau, E., and Bovet, D.: Recherches sur l'action sympathicolytique l'un nouveau dérivé du dioxane. Arch. internat. de pharmacodyn. et de thérap., *46*:178, 1933.
Ganem, E. J., and Cahill, G. F.: Pheochromocytomas coexisting in adrenal gland and retroperitoneal space, with sustained hypertension. New England J. Med., *238*:692, 1948.
Glynn, E. E.: The adrenal cortex, its rests and tumors; its relation to other ductless glands, especially to sex. Quart. J. Med., *5*:157, 1942.
Goldenberg, M.: Adrenal medullary function. Am. J. Med., *10*:627, 1951.
———, Faber, M., Alston, E. J., and Chargaff, E. C.: Evidence for the occurrence of nor-epinephrine in the adrenal medulla. Science, *109*:534, 1949.
———, Snyder, C. H., and Aranow, H., Jr.: New test for hypertension due to circulating epinephrine. J.A.M.A., *135*:971, 1947.
Green, D. M.: Pheochromocytoma and chronic hypertension. J.A.M.A., *131*:1260, 1946.
———, Nelson, J. N., Dobbs, G. A., and Smally, R. E.: Bilateral adrenalectomy in malignant hypertension and diabetes. J.A.M.A., *144*:439, 1950.
Grimson, K. S., Longino, F. H., Kernodle, C. E., and O'Rear, H. B.: Treatment of a patient with a pheochromocytoma. J.A.M.A., *140*:1273, 1949.
Guarneri, V., and Evans, J. A.: Pheochromocytoma: report of a case, with a new diagnostic test. Am. J. Med., *4*:806, 1948.
Hatch, F. N., Richards, V., and Spiegl, R.: Adrenal medullary tumor (pheochromocytoma). Am. J. Med., *6*:633, 1949.
Hyman, A., and Mencher, W. H.: Pheochromocytoma of adrenal gland. J. Urol., *49*:755, 1943.
Kelly, H. M., Piper, M. C., Wilder, R. M., and Walters, W.: Case of paroxysmal hypertension with paraganglioma of right suprarenal gland. Proc. Staff Meet., Mayo Clinic, *11*:65, 1936.
Kenyon, A. T.: Adrenal cortical tumors, physiologic considerations; in Endocrinology of Neoplastic Diseases. New York, Oxford University Press, 1947, p. 245.
———: Adrenal cortical tumors: physiologic considerations. Surgery, *16*:194, 1944.
Kepler, E. J., and Keating, F. R.: Diseases of the adrenal glands. II. Tumors of the adrenal cortex, diseases of the adrenal medulla and allied disturbances. Arch. Int. Med., *68*:1010, 1941.
———, Sprague, R. G., Mason, H. L., and Power, M. H.: The pathologic physiology of adrenal cortical tumors and Cushing's syndrome. Recent Progr. Hormone Research, *2*:345, 1948.

Kepler, E. J., and Mason, H. L.: Relation of urinary steroids to the diagnosis of adrenal cortical tumors and adrenal cortical hyperplasia; quantitative and isolation studies. J. Clin. Endocrinol., 7:543, 1947.

Labbé, M., Tinel, J., and Doumer: Crises solaires et hypertension paroxystique en rapport avec une tumeur surrénale. Bull. et mém. Soc. méd. d. hôp. de Paris, 46: 982, 1922.

LaDue, J. S., Murison, P. J., and Pack, G. T.: The use of tetraethylammonium bromide as a diagnostic test for pheochromocytoma. Ann. Int. Med., 29:914, 1948.

Laubry, C.: Hypertension paroxystique quérie par la radiothérapie de la region surrénale. Bull. et mém. Soc. med. d. hôp. de Paris, 51:1216, 1927.

Lisser, H.: Case of adrenal cortical tumors in adult male causing gynecomastia and lactation. Endocrinology, 20:567, 1936.

Lowenstein, B. E., Corcoran, A. C., and Page, I. H.: Determination of corticosteroids in urine. Endocrinology, 39:82, 1946.

Lukens, F. D. W.: Diagnosis and treatment of cortical tumors. M. Clin. North America, 26:1803, 1942.

———, Flippin, H. F., and Thigpin, F. M.: Adrenal cortical adenoma with absence of the opposite adrenal. Am. J. M. Sc., 193:812, 1937.

McCullagh, E. P., and Engel, W. J.: Pheochromocytoma with hypermetabolism; report of two cases. Ann. Surg., 116:61, 1942.

MacKeith, R.: Adrenal-sympathetic syndrome; chromaffin tissue tumor with paroxysmal hypertension. Brit. Heart J., 6:1, 1944.

Maier, H. C.: Intrathoracic pheochromocytoma. Ann. Surg., 130:1059, 1949.

Manasse, P.: Ueber die hyperplastichen Tumoren der Nebennieren. Virchows Arch. f. path. Anat., 133:391, 1893.

Mayo, C. H.: Paroxysmal hypertension with tumor of retroperitoneal nerve: report of a case. J.A.M.A., 89:1047, 1927.

Phillips, B.: Intrathoracic pheochromocytoma. Arch. Path., 30:916, 1940.

Pincoffs, M. C.: A case of paroxysmal hypertension associated with suprarenal tumor. Tr. A. Am. Physicians, 44:295, 1929.

Prohaska, J. V., Harms, H. P., and Dragstedt, L. R.: Epinephrine hypertension. Ann. Surg., 106:857, 1937.

Roth, G. M., and Kvale, W. F.: A tentative test for the diagnosis of pheochromocytoma. J. Lab. & Clin. Med., 30:366, 1945.

Soffer, L. J.: Diseases of the Adrenals. Philadelphia, Lea & Febiger, 1948.

Spear, H. C., and Griswold, D.: The use of dibenamine in pheochromocytoma. New England J. Med., 239:736, 1948.

Sprague, R. G., Kepler, E. J., Keating, F. R., Jr., and Power, M. H.: Coexisting Addison's disease and diabetes mellitus; comparative effects of compound E (17-hydroxy-11-dehydrocorticosterone) and allied substances in three cases. J. Clin. Investigation, 26:1198, 1947.

Talbot, N. B., Saltzman, A. H., Wixom, R. L., and Wolfe, J. K.: Colorimetric assay of urinary corticoid-like substances. J. Biol. Chem., 160:535, 1945.

Vaquez, H., Donzelot, E., and Gerandel, E.: Les Crises d'hypertension artérielle paroxystique. Presse méd., 34:1329, 1926.

Walters, W., and Kepler, E. J.: Adrenal cortical tumors and their treatment: a study of seven operated cases. Ann. Surg., 107:881, 1938.

——— and Sprague, R. G.: Hyperfunctioning tumors of the adrenal cortex with report of eight cases. Ann. Surg., 129:677, 1949.

———, Wilder, R. M., and Kepler, E. J.: The suprarenal cortical syndrome, with presentation of ten cases. Ann. Surg., 100:690, 1934.

Wells, A. H., and Boman, P. G.: The clinical and pathological identity of pheochromocytoma: report of a case. J.A.M.A., 109:1176, 1937.

Young, H. H.: A technique for the simultaneous exposure and operation on the adrenals. Surg., Gynec. & Obst., 63:179, 1936.

Zintel, H., Wolferth, C. C., Jeffers, W. A., Hafkenschiel, J. H., and Lukens, F. D. W.: Subtotal adrenalectomy in the treatment of patients with severe essential hypertension. Ann. Surg., 134:351, 1951.

CHAPTER 11

THE PITUITARY, THYMUS, AND GONADS

TUMORS OF THE PITUITARY

Various aspects of the physiology of the pituitary gland have been discussed previously in appropriate sections. It remains to consider the nature of certain tumors of this organ.

Eosinophil (Acidophilic) Adenoma of the Anterior Lobe. These neoplasms, which comprise approximately 20 per cent of pituitary adenomas, secrete abnormal amounts of certain of the anterior pituitary hormones. When the tumor arises in pre-adult life before ossification is complete, giantism results. If the tumor develops in an adult the condition known as acromegaly may be produced, characterized by the following changes: (1) overgrowth of the bones of the hands, feet and face; (2) atrophy of the gonads with decline of sexual function (this may be preceded by a temporary increase in sexual function); (3) enlargement of the viscera; (4) stimulation of the thyroid, adrenals and parathyroids, which may result in signs of excessive activity of these organs; and (5) derangements in glucose metabolism.

Basophil Adenoma of the Anterior Pituitary. The hormonal excesses produced by this tumor result in the clinical picture frequently referred to as "Cushing's syndrome." The following features may be present: (1) obesity of the trunk ("buffalo type"); (2) purplish striae over the lower abdomen; (3) cyanosis of the face, hands and feet; (4) pigmentation of the skin and excessive growth of hair ("bearded women"); (5) demineralization of the bones; (6) suppression of sexual function with atrophy of genitalia; and (7) derangement of glucose metabolism.

It will be seen that many of these findings of "pituitary basophilism" are similar to those which accompany adrenocortical tumors, masculinizing tumors of the ovary, and, very rarely, thymic neoplasms. Indeed, at times it may be exceedingly difficult, if not impossible, to determine the location of the lesion. (See Chapter 10 for diagnostic procedures.)

Chromophobe Adenoma. These tumors constitute about 73 per cent of the pituitary adenomas (German) and are by far the largest group of pituitary tumors requiring surgical intervention. The function of the chromophobe cell is unknown, but the symptoms of chromophobe tumors are those of hypopituitarism. Among these are loss of libido in the male and cessation of menstruation in the female. Body hair becomes scant and men need shave only rarely. The basal metabolic rate is usually diminished and obesity may develop.

Pituitary Adamantinomas. These tumors usually occur in childhood and the clinical picture produced results from hypopituitarism and from pressure on surrounding structures. These tumors can usually be differentiated from other pituitary tumors by virtue of the fact that they are frequently associated with calcification which is visible on roentgen examination.

Suprasellar Cyst. This lesion originates in Rathke's pouch and presents a fairly common surgical problem in children. The symptoms and signs vary greatly, depending upon the position of the tumor along the pituitary stalk. If the tumor arises high on this structure, symptoms of increased intracranial pressure may be produced and optic nerve involvement may be present. Since these cysts at times reach relatively enormous size, a number of adjacent structures may be compressed with symptoms appropriate to the areas involved. These tumors arise in the midline but they are predominantly unilateral in position.

Differential Diagnosis of Pituitary Tumors

The clinical picture of acromegaly or giantism may be sufficient to permit a diagnosis of eosinophil adenoma. Patients with these tumors often have severe headaches, but as a rule visual disturbances do not occur until late. The visual defect, when it occurs, is usually that of bitemporal hemianopsia (from pressure on the optic chiasm) or a right or left homonymous hemianopsia. Eventually patients with eosinophil adenomas may exhibit signs of hypopituitarism.

As noted above, the differentiation of basophilic adenomas from tumors of the adrenal cortex, ovary and thymus may be most difficult. The pituitary tumor is not large enough to produce pressure symptoms and thus the optic nerves are not affected. There is usually no calcification in the region of the pituitary, and headaches are not common. Frequently the diagnosis is reached only by the exclusion of lesions elsewhere. Urinary steroid studies should prove increasingly helpful.

The chromophobe adenoma is more readily diagnosed. In the adult the symptoms are those of hypopituitarism without acromegaly or basophilism. Visual disturbances may not appear for years, but when they occur they are most commonly represented by homonymous hemianopsia. Roentgen examination may reveal enlargement of the sella turcica.

Management of Pituitary Tumors

The eosinophil adenoma is best treated initially with deep roentgen therapy. If this has no effect and the tumor progresses, as evidenced by an increasing defect in the visual fields and by headache, surgical intervention is indicated. It is not necessary to remove the entire tumor but the optic chiasm must be freed from pressure. The basophil adenoma is best treated with deep roentgen therapy and practically never requires surgery. The chromophobe adenoma is the most common of these lesions and the treatment is predominantly surgical. "The primary object of the operation is to conserve the vision that is still present, but unless optic atrophy has developed, much of the visual loss may be restored" (Peet). The pituitary adamantinomas and suprasellar cysts should be completely excised where possible.

DISEASES OF THE THYMUS GLAND

Despite repeated efforts over a period of many years it is still impossible to assign definite functions to the thymus, and to assess the precise physiologic significance of abnormalities found in this gland is difficult. Certain lesions of the thymus upon which the surgeon may be asked to render an opinion will be touched upon.

Hyperplasia of the Thymus. At times referred to as status lymphaticus, hyperplasia of the thymus is usually associated with enlargement of lymphatic tissue elsewhere. It was formerly thought to be a common cause of respiratory obstruction in children and was treated by roentgen therapy or surgical excision. However, either the condition has become much less common or the diagnosis has often been made erroneously in the past. The writer has never seen a case that required therapy, but ACTH therapy would probably effect a prompt decrease in the size of the thymus if needed.

Malignant Tumors of the Thymus. These are not common, but when they arise the prognosis is poor. These lesions may run the gamut of the lymphatic potentialities. Carcinoma may arise in the epithelium of Hassall's corpuscles, and various types of sarcomas and teratomas have been reported. However, lymphosarcoma appears to be the most commonly diagnosed tumor. Roentgen therapy is preferable to surgery, but neither is often curative.

Benign Tumors of the Thymus. These are of interest chiefly because of the frequency with which they are associated with myasthenia gravis. In 1941 Blalock and his associates suggested thymectomy as a treatment for this incompletely understood neuromuscular disease on the basis of the fact that in almost one-half the cases reported in the literature a thymic tumor had been found. Sufficient time has now elapsed to permit certain tentative conclusions concerning the value of thymectomy in this condition. Improvement has been observed in a considerable number of those patients in whom a tumor was found and removed at operation, but the removal of a tumor is not always followed by a remission of the disease. Patients whose thymus harbors no tumor are much less likely to be benefited by operation. To complicate the picture, spontaneous remissions are common in this disease, and it is also possible that trauma may stimulate metabolic activity which in itself effects an improvement in the patient's condition. Treatment with ACTH has not proved of significant value.

FUNCTIONING TUMORS OF THE OVARY

Certain functioning tumors of the ovary are of particular importance to the general surgeon by virtue of the fact that they may produce a clinical picture which is difficult to distinguish from that associated with tumors of other endocrine organs.

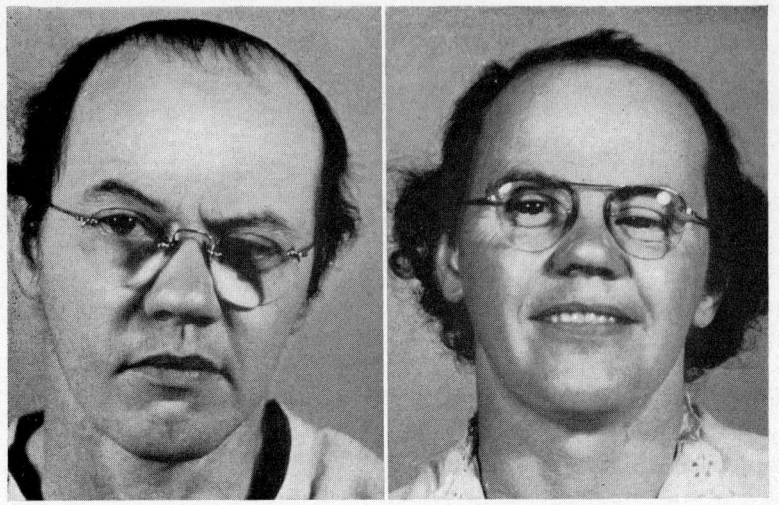

Fig. 43. Preoperative and postoperative appearance of patient with masculinizing adrenal rest of ovary; time interval, five years. (Rhoads, J. E., Zintel, H. A., and Horn, R.: J.A.M.A., in press.)

Masculinizing Tumors. These produce androgenic substances which at first result in amenorrhea, retrogression of the breasts, and occasionally a loss of the subcutaneous fat which gives the female form its contour. This regression from the typical feminine picture is followed by definite masculine characteristics consisting of excessive hair growth on the face and elsewhere, hypertrophy of the clitoris and deepening of the voice. The chief representatives of this group of tumors are the arrhenoblastoma and the adrenal rests.

Feminizing Tumors. These are represented particularly by the granulosa cell tumor, which produces an excess of the estrogens which in normal amounts are responsible for the development of the secondary sex characteristics appropriate to the female. The clinical picture associated with this tumor will vary with the age of the patient. Young girls may exhibit precocious sexual development and premature menses. During menstrual life, however, the normally developed sex characteristics may mask the presence of the feminizing tumor. In postmenopausal women a functioning granulosa cell tumor may cause a resumption of uterine bleeding simulating menstrual periods, but in this age group the breasts have lost their capacity to respond to estrogen stimulation and hence would give no clue to the diagnosis (Novak).

Management of Functioning Ovarian Tumors

The treatment of tumors of this entire group is surgical, but the extent of the operation which should be performed depends to some extent upon the age of the patient (Novak). In young persons, in whom it is most important to preserve reproductive function, the operation should be a conservative one. If no tumor can be found, the ovary should not be removed on the suspicion that it may harbor a minute granulosa cell tumor. There are more common causes of precocious puberty. If a tumor is found, only the adnexa on the involved side should be removed, and postoperative irradiation is obviously contraindicated because of the danger of sterility. Careful follow-up is imperative because of the fact that many of these tumors are malignant.

When such tumors are encountered in older women, the entire adnexa and uterus should be removed. This should be done regardless of whether or not the tumor appears to the operator to be benign, since frequently the diagnosis of malignancy is not made until the microscopic sections have been examined. Although the results with malignant functioning ovarian tumors are somewhat better than those with malignant ovarian tumors in general, recurrences are sufficiently common to emphasize the potentially malignant nature of these lesions. Postoperative irradiation is justified as an additional measure for the prevention of recurrence.

TUMORS OF THE TESTIS

Tumors of the testicles represent 0.57 per cent of all malignant tumors in men and are relatively more common in the undescended than in the normally placed organ (Culver). The *etiology* of such tumors is no more certain than is the etiology of tumors in general. The *pathology* of these neoplasms has emerged somewhat from the confusion existing in the past. Benign neoplasms of the testicle are rare, and thus a very serious view must be taken of any tumor of this organ. It serves clarity to recognize two main groups: (1) mixed tumors or teratomas and (2) pure cell types such as seminomas. The mixed tumors are derived from all three primary germinal layers and in any particular tumor all types of cells may be found. However, usually one cell type predominates and in fact the majority of testicular tumors are teratomatous carcinomas.

Excretion of Hormones by Patients with Testicular Tumors. In 1929 Zondek demonstrated that men with testicular tumors might excrete large quantities of gonadotropic hormone in the urine. This finding has both diagnostic and prognostic importance. It is present in the urine in diagnostic amounts in about 85 per cent of testicular tumors and, in general, the greater the amount of hormone excreted the poorer is the prognosis.

Management of Testicular Tumors

Complete surgical excision is the treatment of choice. Unfortunately, though the superficial location of these tumors facilitates early diagnosis, metastatic spread occurs early by way of the lymphatics and simple orchiectomy results in only 15 per cent of cures (Culver). This figure may be increased to approximately 30 per cent by radical surgery which removes the testicle, cord and retroperitoneal tissue with its lymphatics en masse. Irradiation has not proved curative, but it should be employed following radical surgery. In cases which are inoperable, roentgen or radium therapy may achieve variable degrees of palliation.

REFERENCES

Bell, E. T.: Tumors of thymus. J. Nerv. & Ment. Dis., 45:130, 1917.

Best, C. H., and Taylor, N. B.: The Physiological Basis of Medical Practice. 4th ed. Baltimore, The Williams & Wilkins Company, 1945.

Blalock, A. J.: Thymectomy in treatment of myasthenia gravis; report of 20 cases. J. Thoracic Surg., 13:316, 1944.

———, Harvey, A. McG., Ford, F. R., and Lilienthal, J. L., Jr.: Treatment of myasthenia gravis by removal of thymus gland, preliminary report. J.A.M.A., 117:1529, 1941.

———, Mason, M. F., Morgan, H. J., and Riven, S. S.: Myasthenia gravis and tumors of thymic region: report of case in which tumor was removed. Ann. Surg., 110:544, 1939.

Boyd, W.: Surgical Pathology. 6th ed. Philadelphia, W. B. Saunders Company, 1947.

Culver, H.: Tumors of the testicle; in Christopher, F.: Textbook of Surgery. 5th ed. Philadelphia, W. B. Saunders Company, 1949, p. 1307.

German, W. J.: The endocrine effects of pituitary tumors; in Endocrinology of Neoplastic Diseases. New York, Oxford University Press, 1947, p. 63.

Novak, E.: Ovarian tumors with sex hormone function; in Endocrinology of Neoplastic Diseases. New York, Oxford University Press, 1947, p. 108.

Peet, M. M.: Pituitary tumors; in Christopher, F.: Textbook of Surgery. 4th ed. Philadelphia, W. B. Saunders Company, 1945, p. 345.

Selye, H.: Textbook of Endocrinology. Montreal, Acta Endocrinologica, Université de Montreal, 1947.

Twombley, G. H.: The relationship of hormones to testicular tumors; in Endocrinology of Neoplastic Diseases. New York, Oxford University Press, 1947, p. 228.

Zondek, B.: Versuch einer biologischen (hormonalen) Diagnostik beim malignen Hodentumor. Chirurg., 2:1072, 1930.

INDEX

A

Abnormal fluid deposits. See *Fluid deposits, abnormal*
ACE (adrenocortical extract):
 in adrenocortical insufficiency, 59, 61
 effect of, on fluid volume, 17
  on radiosodium distribution in body tissues, 18
  on serum antibodies, 4
 in homeostasis of sodium, 17
 in resection of adrenocortical tumors, 123 et seq.
Acid phosphatase in carcinoma of prostate, 63
Acidophil (eosinophilic) adenoma, 137
ACTH (adrenocorticotrophic hormone):
 effect of, on allergic conditions, 51, 62
  on blood coagulation, 5
  on burns, 51
  on electrolyte concentration in sweat, 18
  on eosinophil count, 10
  on lymphoid tumors, 53
  on nitrogen balance, 28
  in pneumonia, 51
  on serum antibodies, 4
  on serum level of protein-bound iodine, 8
  on surgical infections, 51
  on vitamin C content of adrenal cortex, 31
 in surgical management of adrenocortical tumors, 124
 secretion of, in stress, 1
  effect of high protein diet on, 33
Adamantinoma of pituitary, 138
Addison's disease:
 adrenal crisis in, compared to thyroid crisis, 8
 effect of DOCA in, 5
 electrolyte metabolism in, 5
 operative risk in, 10
Adenomas:
 acidophil, 137
 basophil, 137
 chromophobe, of pituitary, 137
 islet cell, 112 et seq.
 parathyroid, 104 et seq.
 pituitary, 137 et seq.

Adipokinin, 30
Adrenal cortex:
 activity of, in relation to thyroid activity, 8
 influence of, on body fluid compartments, 16 et seq.
  on electrolytes of sweat, 18
  on eosinophil count, 2
  on gastrointestinal secretion following trauma, 20
  on neoplasia, 53, 65
  on nitrogen mobilization, 28 et seq.
  on postoperative retention of salt and water, 18
  on wound healing, 52
 amorphous fraction of secretion of, in water and salt metabolism, 18
 effect of epinephrine on, 10
 of thiamine deficiency on, 32
 function of, in stress, 2, 3
 hormones of. See also *Adrenal cortex, steroids of*, and *Cortisone*
  effect of, on carbohydrate metabolism, 5, 28, 30
   on kidney, 16
   on nitrogen mobilization in muscle by thyroxine, 8, 28
   on stimulation of cellular oxygen consumption by thyroid, 8
 hypoplasia of, on side opposite tumor, 123
 steroids of, 3, 5. See also *Adrenal cortex, hormones of; Cortisone;* and *DOCA*
  effect of adrenocortical tumor on excretion of, 122
  influence of, on bacterial infections, 4
   on body fluid metabolism, 3
   on clotting process, 5
   on immunologic response, 4
   on sodium excretion in urine, 5
 tumors of, 119
  ACE in surgical management of, 123 et seq.
  ACTH in surgical management of, 124
  adrenal insufficiency following resection of, 123
  adrenalectomy for, 124

INDEX

Adrenal cortex, tumors of, bone age in, 122
 clinical manifestations of, 119
  cortisone in surgical management of, 124
 diagnosis of, 120 et seq.
 effects of, on blood sugar, 122
  on corticoid excretion, 6
 osteoporosis in, 122
 preoperative and postoperative care of, 123 et seq.
 prognosis following resection of, 127
 pulmonary metastasis in, 122
 roentgen examination in, 122
 steroid excretion in, 122
 surgical management of, 123 et seq.
 vitamin C content of, effect of ACTH on, 31
Adrenal glands (see also *Adrenal cortex* and *Adrenal medulla*):
 anatomic features and landmarks of, 126
 surgical considerations of, 119 et seq. See also *Adrenalectomy*
 surgical exposure of, 124
Adrenal hypoplasia. See under *Adrenal cortex*
Adrenal medulla:
 emergency function of, 1
 functioning tumors of, 128 et seq.
  bilateral occurrence of, 133
  chemical tests for, 131 et seq.
  clinical picture of, 130
  complications following resection of, 134
  diagnosis of, 131
  historical considerations of, 128
  incidence of, 129
  paroxysmal attacks in, 130
  pathology of, 129
  simulation of diabetes mellitus by, 130
   of hyperthyroidism by, 130
  surgical management of, 133
Adrenalectomy:
 effect of, on lipid mobilization and deposition in liver, 3
 for adrenocortical tumors, 124
 for essential hypertension, 128
 operative technic for, 124
Adrenocortical extract. See *ACE*
Adrenocortical hormones. See *Adrenal cortex, hormones of,* and *Cortisone*
Adrenocortical insufficiency:
 absolute, anesthesia for surgical patients with, 60
  management of, in surgical patients, 59 et seq.
 body fluid compartments in, 17
 relative, management of, in surgical patients, 60

Adrenocortical insufficiency, relative, test for, 61
 in tuberculous patients, incidence of, 61
 use of ACTH in, 61
 use of ACE in, 59 et seq.
 of cortisone in, 59 et seq.
 of DOCA in, 18, 59 et seq.
Adrenocortical reserve, test of, 10
Adrenocorticotrophic hormone. See *ACTH*
Adrenogenital syndrome, 119
Air embolism during thyroidectomy, 87
Air injection, perirenal, 122
Alarm reaction:
 effect of nutrition on, 32
 glycogen storage in, 30
 hyperglycemia in, 1
 liver function in, 2 et seq.
 outline of, 1
 possible role of fever in, 8
 practical implications of, 9
Alkaline phosphatase in serum in hyperparathyroidism, 104
Allergy, effect of ACTH and cortisone on, 51, 62
Ambulation, early. See *Early ambulation*
Amorphous fraction of adrenocortical secretion, effect of, on water and salt metabolism, 18
Anastomoses, functioning of, effect of malnutrition on, 32
Androgens (see also *Testosterone*):
 effect of, on body fluid distribution, 23
  on nitrogen retention, 5, 66
  on somatic growth, 5
 relation of, to 17-ketosteroids, 6
Anesthesia:
 in adrenocortical insufficiency, 60
 intolerance of fatty liver for, 34
 for thyroidectomy, 84
Anoxia in production of irreversible shock, 24
Anti-anabolism, 27
Antibodies:
 diminished response of, in vitamin deficiency, 34
 serum level of, effect of ACTH on, 4
Antidiuretic hormone of posterior pituitary. See under *Pituitary gland, posterior lobe of*
Antilipotropic substances, 30
Appetite, factors affecting, 35
Ascites:
 etiologic factors in, 22
 failure of liver to inactivate posterior pituitary hormone in, 16
 possible role of kidney in production of, 23
 urinary output in, 23
Axis, pituitary-thyroid-adrenal, 9

INDEX

B

Basal metabolic rate:
  in diagnosis of hyperthyroidism, 75 et seq.
  in starvation, 33
Basophil adenoma, 137
Benzodioxane derivatives in diagnosis of pheochromocytoma, 132
Blood coagulation, effect of adrenocortical secretions on, 5
Blood nitrogen in shock, 23
Blood sugar:
  effects of adrenocortical tumors on, 122
  of cortisone on, 5
  of trauma on, 30
Body fluid compartments:
  effects of androgens and estrogens on, 23
  of DOCA on, 17
  role of adrenocortical hormones in maintenance of, 16 et seq.
Body water, total, deuterium oxide in measurement of, 17
Breast, carcinoma of:
  estrogen therapy in, 65
  testosterone therapy in, 54, 64, 65
Burns, ACTH and cortisone in, 51

C

Calcium:
  metabolism of, during immobilization, 46
  serum level of, effect of, on parathyroid activity, 100
    elevation of, following testosterone administration, 65
    in hyperparathyroidism, 102, 103
    in hypoparathyroidism, 88
  urinary excretion of, in hyperparathyroidism, 104
Calcium gluconate, use of, in hypoparathyroidism, 88, 89
Calories:
  carbohydrate as source of, 36
  fat as source of, 37
  protein as source of, 35 et seq.
  requirements of, in postoperative period, 36
Carbohydrate:
  metabolism of, effect of adrenocortical secretions on, 5, 28, 30
    effect of compound F on, 5
    of cortisone on, 5
    of DOCA on, 5
    of endocrines on, 5, 28, 30 et seq.
    relation of, to water and salt metabolism, 15

Carbohydrate, metabolism of, in shock, 23
  as source of calories, 36
Carcinoma. See under specific organ involved, e.g., *Breast, Prostate gland, Thyroid gland*
Cardiac. See *Heart*
Cardiovascular reflexes:
  effects of starvation on, 34
  and postural hemodynamics, 47
Catabolism, possible role of, in nitrogen metabolism, 27
Catalysts, oxidative, relation of vitamins to, 31, 32
Cervix uteri, carcinoma of, effect of progesterone on, 55, 65
Chloride:
  decrease in blood level of, in early postoperative period, 10
  retention of, with DOCA, 5
  urinary excretion of, following trauma, 3, 18 et seq.
Cholesterol as possible precursor of steroids, 6
Choline, effect of, in prevention of fat deposition in liver, 30, 34
Chromophobe adenoma of pituitary, 137
Cirrhosis, abnormal fluid metabolism in, 22
Clotting process, effects of adrenal cortex steroids on, 5
Compound E. See *Cortisone*
Compound F (17-hydroxycorticosterone):
  effect of, on carbohydrate metabolism, 5
  on sodium excretion in urine, 5
Convalescence:
  definition of, 43
  effect of mental outlook on, 48
  investigation of, 11
Conversion ratio of radioactive iodine, 76, 77
Corticoids:
  differentiation of, from 17-ketosteroids, 6
  effect of, on glycogen reserves, 30
  excretion of, normal, 6
    in presence of adrenocortical tumors, 6
  precursors of, 6
Corticosteroids. See *Corticoids*
Cortisone (compound E):
  effect of, on allergic conditions, 51, 62
    on bacterial infections, 4
    on blood sugar, 5
    on carbohydrate metabolism, 5
    on clotting and bleeding time, 5
    on lymphoid tumors, 65
    on nitrogen balance, 28
    on pneumonia, 51

Cortisone (compound E), effect of, on protein-bound iodine level of serum, 8
  on water and salt metabolism, 5
  use of, in adrenocortical insufficiency, 59 et seq.
    in burns, 51
    following removal of adrenocortical tumors, 123 et seq.
    in surgical infection, 51
    in surgical management of adrenocortical tumors, 124
Craniopharyngioma. See *Adamantinoma of pituitary*
Cushing's syndrome, 119. See also *Adrenocortical tumors; Ovary, masculinizing tumors of;* and *Pituitary gland, tumors of*
Cyst:
  suprasellar, 138
  thyroglossal, 70
Cytochrome C in oxygen utilization, 7

D

Decubiti, effect of malnutrition on, 32
11 - Dehydro - 17 - hydroxycorticosterone. See *Cortisone*
Desoxycorticosterone. See DOCA
Deuterium oxide:
  for measurement of total body water, 17
  as tracer in study of fatty acid metabolism, 1
Diabetes insipidus:
  pitressin in treatment of, 66
  thyroid gland in maintenance of, 16
Diabetes mellitus:
  management of, in surgical patients, 62 et seq.
  simulated by functioning tumor of adrenal medulla, 130
Diabetic coma, 63
Dibenamine in test for pheochromocytoma, 132
Diet (see also *Nutrition*):
  effect of, on composition of fats, 29
  protein-rich, effect of, on secretion of ACTH in stress, 33
  psychologic effect of appearance of, 35
  route of administration of, 35
DOCA (desoxycorticosterone):
  effect of, in Addison's disease, 5
  on adrenocortical insufficiency, 18, 60
  on body fluid compartments, 17
  on carbohydrate metabolism, 5
  on chloride retention, 5
  on electrolyte concentration in sweat, 18
  on potassium excretion, 18

DOCA (desoxycorticosterone), effect of, on water retention, 5
  and sodium homeostasis, 18
Dynamic state of body constituents, 1

E

Early ambulation:
  gastro-intestinal function in, 45
  phlebothrombosis in, incidence of, 45
  pulmonary embolism in, incidence of, 45
  wound healing in, 44
Electrolytes:
  metabolism of, in Addison's disease, 5. See also *Fluids and electrolytes, metabolism of*
  of serum, abnormalities of, in presence of adrenocortical tumors, 122
    effect of trauma on, 10
  of sweat, effect of ACTH on, 18
    of DOCA on, 18
    of trauma on, 18
  of urine, effect of operation on excretion of, 18
Emotions, effect of, on convalescence, 48
Endocrines (see also *Hormones* and names of specific secretions):
  effect of, on carbohydrate metabolism, 5, 28, 30
    on fluid and electrolyte metabolism, 15 et seq.
    on neoplasia, 53
    on nitrogen metabolism, 27
  relation of, to vitamins, 31
  therapeutic uses in surgical patients, 59 et seq.
Enzymes:
  effect of hormones on, 8
  nature of, 9
Eosinophilic adenoma, 137
Eosinophils:
  effect of ACTH on total count of, 10
    of adrenal cortex activity on total count of, 2
    of epinephrine on total count of, 10
    of trauma on total count of, 2
Epinephrine:
  effect of, on adrenocortical activity, 1, 10
    on anterior pituitary secretions, 1
    on eosinophil count in pituitary insufficiency, 10
    on iodine discharge from thyroid gland in rats, 7
    on thyroid activity, 1
    on thyrotrophic hormone, 7
  release of, in response to trauma, 1
  subnormal reaction of hypothyroid heart to, 7

INDEX

Estrogens:
  effects of, on neoplasia, 54
    on fluid and salt retention, 65
  role of liver in inactivation of, 34
  use of, in breast carcinoma, 65
    in prostatic carcinoma, 64
Etamon as test for pheochromocytoma, 132
Exophthalmus in hyperthyroidism, 75

F

Fats (see also *Fatty acids*):
  as source of calories, 37
  antilipotropic factors in distribution of, 30
  deposition of, 29
  effect of choline on liver content of, 30, 34
    of diet on composition of, 29
    of lipotropic substances on distribution of, 30
  intravenous preparations of, 37
  in liver, relation of, to tolerance for anesthesia, 29, 34
  mobilization and deposition of, in liver, effect of adrenalectomy on, 3
  in starvation, 34
  thyroid gland in, 30
Fatty acids (see also *Fats*):
  metabolism of, deuterium as tracer in study of, 1
  thiamine in, 32
Feminizing syndrome, 119
Fever:
  effect of, on nutritional requirements, 36
  possible role of, in alarm response, 8
Fluid deposits:
  abnormal, 22 et seq.
    in estrogen therapy, 65
    in testosterone therapy, 65
  effect of testosterone on, 65
Fluids and electrolytes:
  metabolism of, 3
    adrenal cortex in, 3, 5, 16 et seq.
    effect of cortisone on, 5
      of endocrine system on, 15 et seq.
      of insulin on, 15
    following operation, 18 et seq.
Fluid replacement therapy, 21
Fluid volume, effect of ACE on, 17
Foramen caecum, 70

G

Gastrectomy, total, effect of, on appetite, 35

Gastric emptying time, effect of malnutrition on, 32
Gastro-intestinal function in early ambulation, 45
Gastro-intestinal secretions, effect of trauma on, 20
Glucocorticoids, effect of, on glycogen reserves, 30. See also *Corticoids*
Glucose, metabolism of:
  adrenal cortex in, 3
  insulin in, 30
  thyroxine in, 30
Glycogen:
  content in hyperthyroidism, 31
  effect of alarm syndrome on storage of, 30
  of glucocorticoids on storage of, 30
Glycosuria in hyperthyroidism, 31
Goiter:
  nontoxic diffuse, management of, 72
  nontoxic nodular, 73
  toxic, management of, 78. See also *Hyperthyroidism*
Graves' disease. See *Hyperthyroidism*
Growth, somatic, effect of androgens on, 5
Gynecomastia in presence of deranged hepatic function, 34

H

Hashimoto's struma, 95
Heart:
  arrest of, during thyroidectomy, 86, 88
  effect of immobilization on function of, 44
  of thyroxine on function of, 72
  response of, to epinephrine in myxedema, 7
Hepatic. See *Liver*
Hexokinase reaction, effect of insulin on, 9
Histamine test in diagnosis of pheochromocytoma, 131
Homeostasis of sodium, effect of ACE on, 17
Hormones (see also under specific hormones and specific organs):
  effects of, on enzymes, 8
    on tissue repair and regeneration, 52 et seq.
  mechanism of action of, 8
  relation of, to vitamins, 31 et seq.
Hydrogen, transport of, nicotinic acid and riboflavin in, 31, 32
17-Hydroxycorticosterone. See *Compound F*
Hyperglycemia in alarm syndrome, 1
Hyperinsulinism:
  diagnosis of, 113 et seq.

Hyperinsulinism, organic, surgical management of, 115
  prognosis in, following removal of islet cell adenoma, 116
Hyperparathyroidism:
  calcium excretion in, 104
  historical background of, 99
  incidence of, 99
  primary, 100
    management of, 104
    prognosis in, following removal of functioning adenoma, 108
  renal stones in, 99, 102, 103
  secondary, 101
  serum calcium level in, 102
  serum phosphorus level in, 88, 89, 104
Hypertension, essential, adrenalectomy for, 128
Hyperthyroidism:
  diagnosis of, 75 et seq.
  etiology of, 75
  exophthalmus in, 75
  glycosuria in, 31
  I^{131} uptake in, as treatment, 80 et seq.
  laboratory tests for, 75 et seq.
  liver glycogen content in, 31
  management of, 78 et seq. See also *Thyroidectomy*
  radioactive iodine in treatment of, 80 et seq.
    comparison of thyroidectomy and, 79
    simulated by functioning tumor of adrenal medulla (pheochromocytoma), 129, 130
  symptomatology of, 75
  thyroidectomy for. See *Thyroidectomy*
Hypocalcemia:
  following thyroidectomy, 88, 89
  vitamin D in, 89
Hypochloremia, postoperative, 10
Hypoglycemia, causes of, 114
Hypokalemia following trauma, 11
Hypoparathyroid tetany following thyroidectomy, 88, 89
Hypoparathyroidism:
  management of, following thyroidectomy, 88, 89
  serum calcium level in, 88
  serum phosphorus level in, 88
Hypothyroidism. See *Myxedema*

I

I^{131}. See *Iodine, radioactive*
Immobilization:
  effects of, on calcium metabolism, 46
    on cardiac function, 44
    on gastro-intestinal function, 45

Immobilization, effects of, on incidence of phlebothrombosis, 45
  of pulmonary embolism, 45
  of renal stones, 46
  on mental outlook, 48
  on metabolism, 45 et seq.
  on muscle size and strength, 46
  on nitrogen balance, 45
  on postural hemodynamics, 47
  on pulmonary function, 44
  on wound healing, 44
Immunologic response, effect of adrenocortical steroids on, 4
Infections:
  ACTH in, 51
  antibody response in, effects of nutritional deficiencies on, 34
  bacterial, effects of adrenal cortex steroids on, 4
  cortisone in, 51
  effect of malnutrition on, 32
Insulin:
  effect of, on glucose utilization, 30
    on hexokinase reaction, 9
    on water metabolism, 15
  excessive secretion of, by islet cell tumors, 111 et seq.
  relation of, to thiamine, 32
    to vitamin C, 31
Iodine:
  effect of ACTH on protein-bound fraction of serum, 8
  metabolism of, effect of trauma on, 7
  protein-bound, effect of cortisone on serum level of, 8
    of trauma on, 8
  as indicator of thyroid activity, 76
  radioactive, conversion ratio of, 76, 77
    as tracer element, 7
    in treatment of hyperthyroidism, 79 et seq.
    of thyroid metastases, 94
  urinary excretion of, following trauma, 7
Islands of Langerhans:
  historical considerations of, 111
  pathology of, 112
  tumors of, 111 et seq.
    surgical treatment of, 115 et seq.
Islet cell tumors, 111 et seq.

K

17-Ketosteroids (see also *Androgens*):
  and corticoids, differentiation between, 6
  excretion of, in malnutrition, 32
  normal, 6
  pathologic, 6
  precursors of, 6

INDEX

17-Ketosteroids, relation of, to testosterone, 6
Kidney:
  effect of adrenocortical hormones on, 16
    of posterior pituitary antidiuretic hormone on, 16
  possible role of, in ascites, 23
  potassium excretion by, effect of DOCA on, 18
  sodium chloride excretion by, effect of surgical procedures on, 10
  stones in hyperparathyroidism, 99, 102, 103
    incidence of, effect of immobilization on, 46
  urinary function of, effect of major surgery on, 18
  VEM production by, 24

L

Lateral aberrant thyroid, malignant nature of, 94
Lipids See *Fats*
Lipotropic substance, 30
Liver:
  effects of nutrition on, 34
    of qualitative protein deficiency on, 34
  fat content of, effect of choline on, 30, 34
    relation of, to tolerance for anesthesia, 34
  function in alarm syndrome, 2 et seq.
  glycogen content of, in hyperthyroidism, 31
    reserves in, role of glucocorticoids in, 30
    storage in, effect of cortisone on, 5
  inactivation of estrogen by, failure in, 34
    of posterior pituitary antidiuretic hormone by, 16, 22, 34
  lipid deposition in, effect of adrenalectomy on, 3
  role of, in prevention of irreversible shock, 24
Lymph nodes, nitrogen mobilization in, 28
Lymphoid tumors, effect of ACTH on, 65

M

Malignancy (see also *Neoplasia*):
  hormonal therapy in, 63 et seq. See also under names of specific organs and specific hormones

Malnutrition (see also *Starvation*):
  effect of, on alarm response, 10
    on liver function, 34
    on response to surgery, 32
  17-ketosteroid excretion in, 32
  wound healing in, 32
Mecholyl in test for pheochromocytoma, 132
Mental outlook:
  effect of nutrition on, 35
    of prolonged immobilization on, 48
Metabolism (see also under names of specific substances, e.g., *Calcium, Carbohydrate*):
  alterations in, following fracture of long bones, 1
  effects of prolonged immobilization on, 45
  in shock, 23 et seq.
Muscles:
  effects of immobilization on, 46
    of nutrition on strength of, 35
    of thyroid on mobilization of nitrogen in, 8, 28
Myasthenia gravis and tumors of the thymus, 139
Myxedema:
  abnormal fluid deposits in, 23
  following thyroidectomy, 90
  operative risk in, 10, 33

N

Neoplasia, role of endocrines in, 53 et seq. See also under names of specific organs
Nephrolithiasis:
  occurrence of, during bed rest, 46
  in hyperparathyroidism, 103
Nerves, recurrent laryngeal, injury to, during thyroidectomy, 87
Nicotinic acid, role of, in hydrogen transport, 31, 32
Nitrogen:
  balance, effect of ACTH and cortisone on, 28
    of immobilization on, 45
    of injury on, 9, 27 et seq.
  blood urea content of, in shock, 23
  excretion of, effect of testosterone on, 28, 66
    thyroid gland in, 28
  metabolism of, effects of endocrines on, 27 et seq.
    of immobilization on, 45
  mobilization of, adrenocortical hormone in, 28
    in muscle, 8, 28
  retention of, effect of androgens on, 5, 66

Nutrition:
    effect of, on alarm response, 32 et seq.
        on emotional outlook, 35
        on hepatic function, 34
        on muscular strength, 35
        on postural hemodynamics, 34, 47
    requirements of, effect of fever on, 36

O

Osteoporosis in adrenocortical tumors, 122
Ovary, tumors of, 140 et seq.
Oxidative catalysts, relation of vitamins to, 31, 32
Oxygen consumption:
    cellular, effect of adrenocortical hormones on, 8
    of thyroxine on, 7
    Cytochrome C in, 7

P

Pancreas:
    insulin content of, relationship of, to vitamin C, 31
    tumors of, 111
Panhypopituitarism, operative risk in, 10
Parathormone:
    in hypoparathyroidism, 89
    mode of action of, 100
Parathyroid glands:
    adenomas of, 104 et seq.
        operative considerations in, 104 et seq.
    anatomy of, 71, 104 et seq.
    pathologic lesions of, 100
    primary hyperfunction of, 100
    regulation of activity of, 99
    removal of, during thyroidectomy, 88
    secondary hyperfunction of, 101
P.B.I. See *Iodine, protein-bound*
Perirenal air injection, 122
Pheochromocytoma. See *Adrenal medulla, functioning tumors of*
Phlebothrombosis, incidence of, in early ambulation, 45
Phosphatase:
    acid, in carcinoma of prostate, 63
    alkaline, in serum in hyperparathyroidism, 104
Phosphorus:
    serum level of, in hyperparathyroidism, 104
    in hypoparathyroidism, 88, 89
Pitocin, use of, to stimulate uterine contractions, 66
Pitressin in treatment of diabetes insipidus, 66

Pituitary gland:
    anterior lobe of, adenomas of, 137 et seq.
        diuretic action of, 16
        effect of epinephrine on, 1
        in fat mobilization in starvation, 30
        growth hormone of, 52
        in response to trauma, 1
    effects of, on neoplasia, 53
    posterior lobe of, antidiuretic hormone of, 16, 22, 34
        extract of, therapeutic uses of, 66
    suprasellar cyst of, 138
    tumors of, 137 et seq.
    in water and salt metabolism, 16
Pituitary-thyroid-adrenal axis, 9
Plasma volume in starvation, 34
Pneumonia, effect of ACTH and cortisone in, 51
Postural hemodynamics:
    effects of immobilization on, 47
    of nutrition on, 34, 47
Potassium:
    radioactive, in measurement of potassium pool, 17
    serum level of, following trauma, 11
    urinary excretion of, effect of DOCA on, 18
        effect of trauma on, 4, 18
Progesterone, effect of, on carcinoma of uterine cervix, 55, 65
Prostate gland:
    carcinoma of, acid phosphatase in, 63
        effect of stilbestrol in, 64
        of testosterone on, 54, 64
Protein:
    deficiency of, effect of, on circulating antibodies, 34
    effect of diet rich in, on ACTH secretion, 33
    metabolism of, in stress, 27
        role of adrenal cortex in, 3
    postoperative administration of, 35 et seq.
    qualitative deficiency of, effect of, on liver, 34
    as source of calories, 35 et seq.
Protein-bound iodine. See *Iodine, protein-bound*
Pulmonary embolism, incidence of, in early ambulation, 45
Pulmonary function, effect of early ambulation on, 44

R

Radioiodine. See *Iodine, radioactive*
Radiosodium. See *Sodium, radioactive*
Recurrent laryngeal nerves, injury to, during thyroidectomy, 87

INDEX

Renal. See *Kidney*
Repair and regeneration of tissues. See *Wound healing*
Respiratory obstruction during and following thyroidectomy, 89
Riboflavin, role of, in hydrogen transport, 31, 32
Riedel's struma, 95

S

Salts (see also *Electrolytes*):
  metabolism of, effect of amorphous fraction of adrenal cortex secretion on, 18. See also *Fluids and electrolytes, metabolism of*
  postoperative retention of, effect of adrenocortical activity on, 18
Serum antibodies, effect of adrenocortical secretions on, 4
Shock:
  blood urea nitrogen in, 23
  metabolism in, 23 et seq.
Sodium:
  excretion of, in urine, effect of adrenocortical steroids on, 5
    following trauma, 3, 10, 19
    in sweat, 18
  homeostasis of, effect of ACE in, 17
    of DOCA in, 18
  radioactive, effect of adrenocortical steroids on distribution of, 18
    in measurement of sodium pool, 17
Spleen in alarm response, 1
Starvation (see also *Malnutrition*):
  effect of, on basal metabolic rate, 33
    on cardiovascular reflexes, 34
    on plasma volume, 34
  fat mobilization in, 30
Steroids. See under specific organs and specific compounds
Stilbestrol, use of, in prostatic carcinoma, 64
Stress. See *Alarm reaction* and *Trauma*
Struma lymphomatosa, 95
Suprasellar cyst, 138
Sweat:
  electrolytes of, effect of ACTH on, 18
    of adrenocortical secretions on, 18
    of DOCA on concentration of, 18
    of trauma on, 18
Sympathicolytic agents, 131, 132

T

Testicles, tumors of, 141 et seq.
Testosterone:
  effect of, on carcinoma of the breast, 54, 64, 65
    of the prostate, 54, 64
  effect of, on fluid deposits, 65
    on nitrogen balance, 28, 66
    on serum calcium level, 65
  relation of, to 17-ketosteroids, 6
Tetany, hypoparathyroid:
  following thyroidectomy, 88, 89
  vitamin D in, 89
Tetraethylammonium salts as test for pheochromocytoma, 132
Thiamine:
  as coenzyme in fatty acid metabolism, 32
  deficiency of, effect of, on adrenal cortex, 32
  relationship of, with insulin, 32
Thiouracil, effect of, on I^{131} uptake of thyroid metastases, 94
Thymus gland, diseases of, 139
Thyroglossal cyst, 70
Thyroid gland:
  activity of, effect of epinephrine on, 1
    protein-bound iodine level as indicator of, 76
    relation of, to adrenocortical activity, 8
  anatomy of, 69
  carcinoma of, 90 et seq.
  in diabetes insipidus, 16
  effect of, on neoplasia in rats, 53
    on nitrogen excretion, 28
    on repair and regeneration of tissue, 52
  embryology of, 69
  in fat metabolism, 30
  lateral aberrant, malignant nature of, 94
  metastases of, radioactive iodine in treatment of, 94
  operative removal of. See *Thyroidectomy*
  pathology of, 72
  physiology of, 71
  possible function of, in stress, 1, 7
Thyroid stimulating hormone. See *TSH*
Thyroidectomy:
  air embolism during, 87
  anesthesia for, 84
  cardiac arrest during, 86, 88
  complications of, 85 et seq.
  effect of, on I^{131} uptake by thyroid metastases, 94
  hemorrhage in, 86, 90
  hypocalcemia following, 88
  myxedema following, 90
  operative technic of, 82 et seq.
  recurrent-laryngeal-nerve injury during, 87
  removal of parathyroid glands during, 88

Thyroidectomy, respiratory obstruction during and following, 89
  subtotal, preoperative and postoperative care in, 81 et seq.
  as treatment for hyperthyroidism, comparison of, with I^{131}, 79 et seq.
Thyroiditis, chronic ligneous, 95
Thyrotropin. See TSH
Thyroxine:
  diuretic effect of, 16
  effect of, on cellular oxygen consumption, 7
    on heart muscle, 72
  in glucose metabolism, 30
  in mobilization of nitrogen, 8, 28
  relation of, to adrenocortical hormone, 8, 28
  in vitamin A metabolism, 31
Tissue repair and regeneration. See Wound healing
Trauma:
  adrenal cortex in, 2, 3
  effect of, on ACTH secretion, 1, 33
    on blood sugar, 30
    on chloride excretion in urine, 3, 18 et seq.
    on electrolytes of serum, 10
      of sweat, 18
    on eosinophil count, 2
    on epinephrine release, 1
    on gastro-intestinal secretions, 20
    on iodine excretion in urine, 7
    on iodine metabolism, 7
    on nitrogen balance, 9, 27 et seq.
    on pituitary gland secretions, 1
    on potassium excretion in urine, 4, 18
    on protein metabolism, 27
    on protein-bound iodine fraction of serum, 8
    on serum potassium level, 11
    on sodium excretion in urine, 3, 10, 18, 19
    on TSH secretion, 7
    on urine volume, 18
    on water and electrolyte excretion in urine, 3, 18
    on water transfer from cells, 11
  thyroid gland in, 1, 7
TSH (thyroid stimulating hormone):
  diuretic effect of, 16
  effect of epinephrine on, 1
    of stress on secretion of, 7
  influence of, on I^{131} uptake by thyroid metastases, 94
Tuberculosis as etiology in adrenocortical insufficiency, 61
Tumors. See under specific organs and specific names, e.g., Adenomas

U

Urine:
  calcium excretion in, in hyperparathyroidism, 104
  chloride excretion in, following trauma, 3, 18 et seq.
  decreased output of, in ascites, 23
    following major surgical procedure, 18
  electrolyte excretion in, effect of operation on, 18
  iodine excretion in, following operation, 7
  17-ketosteroid excretion in, 6
  potassium in excretion, effect of DOCA on, 18
  nitrogen retention in, effect of testosterone on, 66
  sodium excretion in, effect of compound F on, 5
    of trauma on, 3, 10, 18, 19
  steroid excretion in, effect of adrenocortical tumors and hyperplasia on, 122
  water and electrolyte excretion in, in early postoperative period, 3, 18
Uterine cervix, carcinoma of, effect of progesterone on, 55, 65

V

Vaso-depressor material in shock, 24
Vaso-excitatory material in shock, 24
VDM (vaso-depressor material) in shock, 24
VEM (vaso-excitatory material) in shock, 24
Vitamin(s):
  A, metabolism of, thyroxine in, 31
  C content of adrenal cortex, effect of ACTH on, 31
  C deficiency, relation of, to pancreatic insulin content, 31
  D in hypoparathyroid tetany, 89
  deficiency of, effect of, on circulating antibodies, 34
  relation of, to hormones, 31 et seq.
    to oxidative catalysts, 31, 32

W

Water:
  excretion and distribution of, effect of adrenocortical secretions on, 16, 18
  effect of anterior pituitary on, 16
  metabolism of. See Fluids and electrolytes, metabolism of

Water, retention of, following DOCA administration, 5
   following operation, 4, 18
      effect of adrenocortical activity on, 18
   transfer of, from cells, effect of trauma on, 11

Water, urinary excretion of, effect of trauma on, 3, 18

Wound healing:
   effect of adrenocortical hormones on, 52
   of early ambulation on, 44
   of hormones on, 52 et seq.
   of malnutrition on, 32